TERESA SHIEL

SWEET CHANGE

TRUE STORIES OF TRANSFORMATION

"Therefore, if anyone is in Christ, he is a new creation;

old things have passed away; behold,
all things have become new."

2 Corinthians 5:17 NIV

SWEET CHANGE
TRUE STORIES OF TRANSFORMATION

Printed in the USA

ISBN: 978-0-9910012-3-1

Library of Congress Control Number: 2013951297

Published by Write the Vision | Columbia, Missouri

To Contact the Author:

http://teresashieldsparker.com

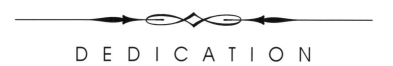

DEDICATION

Dedicated to every caterpillar who longs to be a butterfly.

*May this book be the impetus to propel you forward on the most amazing,
God-directed journey you have ever undertaken.*

*May you find the gold that resides deep inside you
placed by the hand of God.*

*May you experience His grace in a deeper
and more profound way than you ever have before.*

*May you understand what it truly means
to become a new creation in Christ.*

May you learn to soar.

ACKNOWLEDGEMENTS

It's hard to thank everyone who had a part in this book. I want to give special thanks to several who made the process go more smoothly.

Thanks to my family, friends, extended family and staff for supporting me, loving me and putting up with me through everything I neglected for the season of writing this book.

Thanks so much to my diligent first readers: Charlie Warren, Marilyn Logan, Lucie Winborne and Judy English. I can't thank you enough for your labor of love.

To my prayer group: I felt your prayers, every one of them, especially through the times it seemed impossible for this book to ever get written, edited, designed and published in less than four months.

A very special thanks to those who contributed their stories for this book: Russ Hardesty, Rhonda Burrows, Lindsey Summers, Judy English, Mark Randall Shields, Pam Leverett, Sundi Jo Graham, Andrew Parker, Donna Falcioni Barr, Anastacia Maness, Kimberly Weger, Ronda Pickett Waltman, Nora Ann Treguboff Saggese, Aida Ingram, Tom Graddy, Heather Tucker and Mindy Nave.

Thanks also to the wonderful Wendy K. Walters for the cover design. She also designed the cover of *Sweet Grace* so it was great to have a design with the same look and feel. A special thanks to my son, Andrew Parker, for helping format the interior pages and answering all my computer emergencies. Thanks to Roy Parker for supporting me as only he can.

Above all, thanks to the Great I Am, my Lord and Master, the only One who can orchestrate the sweetest change of all.

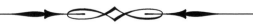

C O N T E N T S

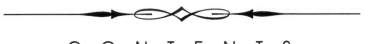

C O N T E N T S

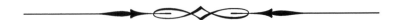

"Do not be conformed to this world, this age, fashioned after and adapted to its external, superficial customs, but be transformed, changed, by the entire renewal of your mind, by its new ideals and its new attitude, so that you may prove for yourselves what is the good and acceptable and perfect will of God, even the thing which is good and acceptable and perfect in His sight for you.

Romans 12:1-2 AMP

AUTHOR'S NOTE

The moment of change for those who have stubborn weight issues is a difficult concept to grasp. How can you be eating everything you desire one moment and the next second make a decision that will change your life?

It's obviously not as easy as that. However, nothing worth having ever comes easy. Weight, whether it is 20 pounds or 220 pounds, is not easy to lose. It's easy to put it on, but oh so difficult to take off.

Still, there is a moment in time when things shift and everything becomes different. One moment I was eating everything I craved or wanted and the next I made a decision and headed towards health.

I really never thought I would reach the moment of change. I knew others had, but I figured I was a hopeless case. After it happened to me, I recognized it as the key to becoming healthy, breaking free of addiction, losing weight and keeping it off.

I also knew there are a lot of other ingredients that go into the weight loss soup mix. So I wrote my weight loss memoir *Sweet Grace: How I Lost 250 Pounds*, in 2013. Along with it I developed the *Sweet Grace Study Guide* to help folks take the journey themselves.

Yet, the key piece of the moment of change still seemed to baffle folks. I knew several months after *Sweet Grace* was released that I would write another book about the change process. Wrapping my brain around how to do that took another nine months or more. Yes, just like having a baby. What people really wanted to know was how they could have their own moment of change.

What causes one person to change his or her mindset and lifestyle is different from that of another person. It's not a one-size-fits-all diagram. How could I share a step-by-step plan then? The answer came as I started the Sweet Change Weight Loss Coaching Group. Those in the group were experiencing change, but each one's change moment was different. Why and how each person made the decision was as unique as they were.

TRUE STORIES

Change motivators, such as being told one only has five years to live, might not be as life-changing to an individual as a two-year-old's frank observation that his grandpa is fat. I began to realize stories of others' change moments and transformations are great inspiration for others.

So why not let people tell their change stories? I already knew several who had lost over 100 pounds. I would invite them and others to share their stories. Connecting them would be material regarding various aspects of change that I have experienced.

I began contacting people, running into people, remembering people and being led to people who had a story of transformation. To my delight, almost everyone I invited agreed to participate in this project.

The stories range from Sundi Jo Graham, who has lost 145 pounds, to those whose loss ranges from 20 to 109 pounds. Judy English, who lost weight 30 years ago, is still on her journey. Mindy Nave is just starting hers. Their ages range from Russ Hardesty, in his 70s, to Lindsey Summers, who is 20. Some have had issues with both alcohol and food. Some are bonafide sugar addicts while others have learned how to allow themselves to eat only small portions of things with sugar.

> Each person's moment of change is unique and different.

The moments of change for some had to do with food allergies or other health issues. Other change work happened because the reality hit home they might not be around to see their children or grandchildren grow up. Some simply needed education and training about how to eat for optimal health. Some finally discovered a way of moving that was fun for them. One thing is common for all: they are discovering and implementing a totally new way of thinking and living.

When you finish reading *Sweet Change*, you will have met 18 ordinary people (including me) who have turned around and headed towards health. These are men and women, young and old, who are busy living their lives just like you. In other words, they are people to whom you can relate.

I know these individuals will inspire you as they have me. Their stories are examples of how God can work in any situation and circumstance to bring deliverance from addictions.

In each chapter you will find information from me at the beginning and a personal change story written by one of the others. The first chapter includes my change story as well and some additional information.

At the back of the book, you will find a final chapter from me, photos of those featured in the book, how to get additional resources and how to stay in touch with me.

Let's get started on the Sweet Change journey.

— Teresa Shields Parker

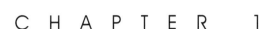

BECOMING A BUTTERFLY

P robably the sweetest change in nature is that of the metamorphosis into a butterfly. The change is indeed transformational, from a crawling worm-like insect to a beautiful creature that can fly.

The sweetness of a butterfly, like the flowers it pollinates, seems to be to add beauty and uniqueness to the world around it. What a wonderful purpose. In essence, that should be our purpose. We should endeavor to bring some kind of beauty or positive energy to the world around us.

Although people are not butterflies, I'm convinced God designed the butterfly's metamorphosis as a parable for our lives. From the time we are born, we have the ability to become something strikingly beautiful in God's plan. It may take us a while to get there, but if we stay true to our design we will.

SUBMIT TO THE PROCESS

In metamorphosis, everything we think we must have to live ceases to exist. Only what God deems necessary remains. Our transformed state was always in God's design for us, a part of our very cells planned before we were born.[1] This total rewiring of our makeup does not take God by surprise. The only intrigue is how long it took us to start the process that results in our transformation.

The process of change seems terrifying when we think about it, but necessary if we really want to transform and not merely change out of our caterpillar suits and put on some butterfly wings. Actually shedding skin, allowing our bodies to dissolve, reconstructing new forms, growing wings and flying is more than a simple costume change.

> It's not merely changing out of our caterpillar suits and putting on some butterfly wings.

Ah, but it is so worth it to really become all we were designed to be before we were even born.[16] It's soaring instead of crawling. It's living instead of dying. It's living in abundance instead of merely existing. It's depending on grace instead of works.

Like a butterfly, we start out as caterpillars or worms, as the Bible has described us. A worm in Biblical times represented something harmful. It was what infested anything that was dead and decaying. The picture was not pretty.

God Himself calls Jacob a "lowly worm,"[2] the lowliest of lows. God says we all have sinned and fallen short of His glorious standard.[3] We fail every day. Already it sounds discouraging. We are like caterpillars, crawling around and eating exactly what we prefer. Our view of life is limited to the perspective from ground level. We know little beyond what is going on right in front of us.

We have no clue that residing within us is the ability to change into a being that can soar and see things from God's perspective. The time will come, if we submit to the process, when our entire reason to exist will not just be to eat everything in sight.

A caterpillar has no concept of this. He only exists. The same verse in which God calls Jacob a worm also says this, "Don't be afraid, people of Israel, for I will help you."[4] We are like caterpillars, but all we need is in Him. Every ounce of willpower in the world will not turn a worm into a butterfly. Only God can do that.

CHRYSALIS

Once the caterpillar enters the chrysalis every part of its body melts or dies, except the imaginal cells which hold its intended design. If you're on track with me you have to be thinking of the Biblical example when the apostle Paul said, "My old self has been crucified with Christ. It is no longer I who live, but Christ lives in me."[5]

The chrysalis is symbolic of death to the old and rebirth of the new. This kind of death is not an eradication of all things Monarch, though. It is more a reassembling and reordering into a creature that has an entirely different purpose and perspective than the caterpillar.

Here's my definition of the chrysalis for us as people: the place where God shelters me for a time so a physical change can occur, one He has orchestrated and designed for me from the beginning of time.

In God's time, the butterfly starts to emerge. Struggle is required to complete the escape to freedom. This creature is radically different from the one who went into the chrysalis. Wings begin to fill with fluid and all of a sudden, it instinctively knows to begin to flap and rise above where it once was.

The development of a butterfly is a wild departure from what has been the norm for the caterpillar. Flying is much different from crawling. It reminds me of the radical change that takes place in us when we accept Christ as Savior. "Therefore, if anyone is in Christ, he is a new creation; old things have passed away; behold, all things have become new."[6]

For us as human beings, there can be and should be other ongoing equally extreme transformations. As we get closer and closer to God, we begin to reflect His glory. We are transformed into His image from glory to glory[7] becoming more like Him.

The things in us, which do not reflect His glory, need to die. We go into God's chrysalis to emerge a totally different creation, reassembled into God's design.

> Change and recreation is a revolutionary process, but we have no cause for fear.

Even though change and recreation is a revolutionary process, we have no cause for fear. God is our fortress.[8] He will cover us with His feathers, and under His wings we will take refuge; His truth will be our shield and buckler.[9] We need only trust Him and the process He has designed for us.

The process of change can be overwhelming. There were many times I wanted to crawl out of my chrysalis. However, once inside, it's impossible to stop the process that is far more than just physical.

It is a process that involves every part of who I am — body, soul and spirit. It is a process that is far from being tasteless and bland. It is a sweet change.

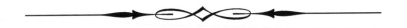

CHANGE STORY
TERESA SHIELDS PARKER

My process of transformation began with changing my twisted mindset of living to eat to one of eating to live. I gave God my wrong attitudes about food and He gave me a new thought process of food being fuel for my body. It was a beautiful exchange that only got better as time went on.

It was hard to deny I had an issue with weight when I was super morbidly obese. I was the queen of denial. I knew I needed to lose weight, but I wanted to lose it and be done with it. Then, I could go back to the way I'd always eaten. I wanted to have my cake (weight loss) and eat it too (anything made with sugar and flour). I couldn't picture my life without eating all the foods I grew up with. They seemed to define me, even as my weight defined me.

I equated my comfort foods with living. If I couldn't eat the things I loved, I felt I couldn't really live. Those foods were my life. They were what I looked forward to. They were what I went to for comfort. They were what I gave others when I wanted to show love.

Eating all those things was severely limiting my life. They were killing me. The real truth of this hit home when I heard Russ Hardesty tell his story of giving up alcohol. I had known Russ for some time. However, I had never heard his story.

He had already had a profound impact on my life through a program called Freedom Seminar. At that seminar I had declared my intention to be a whole, healthy, happy woman. This was a pretty phenomenal statement, since I weighed 430 pounds at the time and was nothing near that description, well except for being a woman.

A light bulb went off somewhere in the recesses of my being.

Although I had done some work towards that, I was far from living my prophetic definition. I knew the exact spot in my bedroom where I placed my secret stash of Starbursts®. I still indulged in every food I wanted. I was still gaining weight faster than the bullet train.

He told told his story of when, why and how he made the choice to give up alcohol. After telling how his life would not be anything near what it is today if he hadn't given up alcohol, he added, almost as an afterthought, "Alcohol is one molecule away from sugar. Alcohol is liquid sugar." These statements stopped me cold and nearly made my heart skip a beat.

A light bulb went off somewhere in the recesses of my being. I knew beyond a shadow of doubt that this was the root of the problem I had tried to solve for over 30 years. And I knew exactly how to fix it.

"I'm like an alcoholic only the addiction is sugar. To lose weight and keep it off I have to stop eating processed sugar," I told myself.

Always before in the back of my mind was the thought that when I lose this weight I will treat myself to a piece or more of my great-grandma's oatmeal cake. I could never eat just one piece of that cake or anything else made with processed sugar and flour. One piece led to more and more and more. What alcoholic can take one drink and leave it alone? I was like that—only the addiction was sugar and it was slowly killing me.

I had diabetes, congestive heart failure, high blood pressure, failing knees and joints and a doctor's proclamation that if I didn't lose weight I'd be dead in five years. I was living like I thought I could beat the odds. In reality, the odds were beating me.

I knew in one second of hearing the words about the connection between alcohol and sugar that my freedom rested in giving up sugar.

"Can sugar be addictive like alcohol?" I asked.

"You can be addicted to anything that controls you," he stated.

> I thought I could beat the odds. In reality, the odds were beating me.

I knew sugar controlled me. I knew I was a sugar addict, even though I had never read a word or done any research about the possibility. I was convicted down to the core of my being. There was no doubt in my mind that every moment of my life had led up to this point. God confirmed what He had been showing me for years.

I thought of a Bible verse I had memorized. "All things are lawful for me, but not all things are profitable. All things are lawful for me, but I will not be mastered by anything."[10] When I memorized it, I didn't understand its significance for me, but in that moment I did. Sugar was not profitable for me. I had to give it up, not for a season, not until I lost a certain amount of weight, but for the rest of my life.

COMFORT FOOD

Suffice it to say, it was not easy giving up what had become my source for comfort — relief of pain, despair, loneliness, frustration, celebration, enjoyment, entertainment and life itself.

I had to realize that life is more than processed sugar and flour. It was hard because all my best childhood memories were tied up in foods made with one or both of those items.

It felt like I was cutting off a part of my legacy by not eating the foods I had gone to for comfort. I would have to put all my eggs in the basket marked Holy Spirit. Would He really come through for me when my emotions were raw and bleeding? Could He comfort me in a better, even more tangible way, than eating two dozen cookies? Did I want to live my life solely for the indulgences I had come to love or was there more to my destiny than being the largest woman anywhere I went?

As a sugar addict, there was no end to the amount of weight I would gain if I continued heading in the same direction. If I mainly ate mainly items made with processed sugar and flour, I would gain weight. It was a fact. However, it was one I had tried to deny and turn a deaf ear to all my life.

From that moment forward, I was cognizant that every step I took was with the intentional mindset — whatever I start now is for the rest of my life. I knew if I decided to turn around and go back to the way I was eating and not moving before, it would mean going back to where I was. I never want to go back there again. It was a prison of my own making.

Each day of this journey, God's grace is the wind at my back propelling me forward. I believe this power of grace activated when He recognized my mind shift. He knows me completely.[11] He knows when I'm being real with my actions and when I'm just roleplaying. Before, I was a really good actress, but I never fooled God. He never chastised me, but He knew I wasn't fully committed.

There was a difference this time. For 30 years with each of the hundreds of diets, programs, potions, pills and magic cures I'd tried, I would say to myself, "Let's dabble in this and see if it works." This time, though, I knew this was the last thing I could try. If this did not work, there was nothing else. I would just have to die a slow death.

> God's grace is the wind at my back propelling me forward.

I knew, and God knew, my entire being had shifted. I felt it move in tandem with my brain. Silently, I prayed, "I am committed to this as a lifestyle change. I can't do it on my own. God, if I ever needed Your help with anything I need it now. I am weak. You are strong.[12] I need Your power. I will surely die without it. I want to live, raise my children, grow old with my husband and serve You. I want to fulfill the destiny You have designed for my life."

When I talk about this moment with others, I call it the moment of change. I believe it's a moment every person must come to. It's the moment the rich, young ruler[13] walked away from, sad and downhearted because Jesus asked him to give up the one thing with which he felt he could never part.

It's really called surrender and God always blesses surrender.

For that young man, it was his money, which had become his identity. Notice for all of eternity this man is called by what was most important to him — rich. For others, it might be alcohol, drugs, cigarettes, an adulterous affair, pornography. It's anything a person puts above God.

For me it was sugar, and eventually gluten. When I laid them down for good, God knew I meant business. It's really called surrender and God always blesses surrender.

Jesus said it this way: "Whoever wants to be My disciple must deny themselves and take up their cross daily and follow Me. For whoever wants to save their life will lose it, but whoever loses their life for Me will save it. What good is it for someone to gain the whole world, and yet lose or forfeit their very self?"[14]

I had done the reverse of this. I had given up absolutely nothing. I had denied myself nothing. I had been trying to hang on to stuff I thought was worth saving, but in the end it would cause me to lose my very soul.

Transformation and abundance go together. When I began the process of change, something magical happened in my life. I discovered the reality that eating the foods I craved does not matter as much as the beauty of everything and everyone around me.

What I thought I craved was just a mirage. Sugar is not the true definition of sweetness. When we say something is sweet, we mean it is the epitome of pleasure. That can only be found in my Lord. When He fulfills my longings, then and only then, does sweetness in its true definition, fill my soul.[15]

His love is deeply intimate, far-reaching, enduring and inclusive. It is endless love beyond measure, beyond academic knowledge. It is extravagant love that pours into me until I am full to overflowing with His greatness.[16] His mighty power within me will bring infinitely more than my greatest request, my most unbelievable dream and exceed my wildest imagination. He will outdo all of these by His miraculous power within me constantly energizing me.[17]

When I gave up and placed every single part of my life, including every desire and craving, in the hands of an almighty Creator, I truly and finally began basking in the abundance of life. I've now lost more than 260 pounds and tons of emotional baggage. I am able to embrace my emotions instead of stuffing them in some deep, dark corner where I think they will never surface. I am able to feel deep love, true compassion and transparent connections with those closet to me.

> I've lost more than 260 pounds and tons of emotional baggage.

My life has changed in so many ways it's hard to describe. In the last year after writing and publishing *Sweet Grace*,[18] my life has exploded with new territories and vistas, new avenues of sharing my story, helping others share their stories and mentoring others who so desperately desire their own lifestyle change.

> I'm living in the place that grace built, a place of abundance, beauty, power, love, victory and freedom.

Now, I'm living in the place that grace built. It's a place of abundance, beauty, power, love, victory and freedom. In this place, there is no room for the lies I used to tell myself. Only truth lives here.

Only truth spoken in love[19] because He wants more than anything for me to have life, overflowing[20] and filled with all the goodness He can pack into it. For so many years I pushed truth away by my wanting, my lustful desire[21] for my lover sugar. It is so ridiculous to trade God for sugar. It is so like God that when I gave Him sugar, He gave me Himself.

Now that's a beautiful exchange.

Teresa Shields Parker is a wife and mother of two grown children. She is an author, coach, speaker and business owner. She enjoys water exercise, reading anything and everything, writing and discovering recipes without processed sugar and gluten. She lives in Columbia, MO.

ENDNOTES

1. Psalm 139:16 NLT
2. Isaiah 41:14 NLT
3. Romans 3:23 NLT
4. Isaiah 41:14 NLT
5. Galatians 2:20 NLT
6. 2 Corinthians 5:17 NKJV
7. 2 Corinthians 3:17-18 NKJV
8. Psalm 91:2 NKJV
9. Psalm 91:4 NKJV
10. 1 Corinthians 6:12 NIV
11. Psalm 139:1-16 NLT
12. 2 Corinthians 12:9-10 NIV
13. Matthew 19:16-26 NIV
14. Luke 9:23-25 NIV
15. Proverbs 13:19 TPT
16. Ephesians 3:19 TPT
17. Ephesians 3:20 TPT
18. *Sweet Grace* is available on Amazon.
19. Ephesians 4:15 NIV
20. John 10:10 AMP
21. James 4:1-7 NIV

SWEET CHANGE

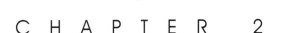

CHAPTER 2

THE CHANGE JOURNEY

A ny change is like going on a journey with ups and downs, twists and turns. It might be said that positive change is a journey where you never really arrive, but only get closer to God.

Change is hard, especially if we have become entrenched in some very unhealthy habits. It is, though, the easiest hard thing I've ever done. It is a journey I will be on until the day I die. Herein lies the problem. As Americans, we want quick, easy change. Put in a dollar and get four quarters right now. However, just because we push the button marked "change" does not mean it will be instantaneous.

COMMITMENT AND DESIRE

Many struggle with commitment and the desire to stay with a change journey for the long haul. It's commitment that makes the difference between those who stay the course and those who stop after the first few weeks.

At the beginning of a weight loss journey, one feels lots of excitement to become different immediately. If the person has 100 pounds to lose, though, quick fixes will not happen. It is only the dedication to a healthy lifestyle change that will keep one on the path.

For any lasting weight loss to occur, changes have to happen on the inside — in one's soul and spirit. They can happen at the same time as exterior changes, but inside change is integral to the process.

Reaching a certain weight should not be the goal as much as making lasting changes in habits. Eating healthy, exercising, embracing your emotions, reaching out to others, being honest and transparent, being connected to God and others are actions that don't just happen overnight. They take time and intentional effort.

> We must take a stand for life in all of its aspects or we will get run over by everything that leads to our death.

A major ingredient in this healthy lifestyle change has to be knowing why we want to lose weight. Most want to live a full and meaningful life. That's really impossible when we can't even get up off the couch, except to make a batch of brownies, of course.

In this fast-paced, push and pull world, we must take a stand for life in all of its aspects or we will get run over by everything that leads to our death. It's interesting that although we say we choose life,[1] when confronted with a choice of something sweet and delectable we know will eventually lead to the destruction of our body, we choose that instead.

God, though, tells us He has plans for our good and not for our disaster.[2] So if His plans are for our good, how did our bodies end up in disaster? It wasn't His choice. Remember, His plan was for our good. Still, He gives us complete freedom to choose. And we chose the course that led to our disaster. It was of our own volition.

WHAT DO I REALLY WANT?

Change is not a one-time choice. It is a moment-by-moment decision about the direction we are headed. It is driven by the overriding want in our lives. For change to be a permanent fixture we have to answer these questions: "What do I want? What kind of person can have what I want?"

When I answered these questions in 1994, I wanted to write books that mattered. I knew I couldn't write those kinds of books unless I was a whole, healthy, happy woman. That meant I was going to have to make some hard choices about giving up some things and replacing them with other things.

This renewal of our minds and the way we think is a transformation — a change. It's a decision, which requires a dedication of our bodies to God. It is sacrificing what we want for what is pleasing to Him.[3]

It wasn't easy. It meant totally giving up the things I craved, never to pick them up again. I'm an all or nothing person, black and white, do or don't. It's how I'm wired. Some call it the personality of an addict.

The idea of denying myself[4] something I loved and living a fasted lifestyle for the rest of my life was an entirely new way of thinking for me. Sure, I knew what the Bible said about denying myself, but I attributed that to giving up Sunday mornings to go to church, not to changing my entire life.

This was not a flippant, fly-by-night decision for me. However, I can define the exact moment of change. I know one moment I was eating my way through bags of candy and the next I gave them up never to visit them again.

Many have asked me, "How long did it take you to give up sugar?" I say, "One second or 61 years, however you want to look at it." Every second of my life leading up to the moment of change was involved in that decision and every second after that and for as long as I live will be, as well. I will be giving it up for the rest of my life in the choices I make moment by moment.

ADDICTION

Abstinence where sugar and gluten are concerned is the only course of action for me. Others may be able to eat a little in moderation. Each person has to know for himself or herself.

Part of that knowing for me was being honest with myself. I grieved just thinking about giving up sugar. That alone told me I was chained, bound, addicted. It was a stronghold I had allowed to take root in my life. For it to be broken I had to allow God to help me give it up completely.

The part of me that doesn't like to be captive hated the idea that I was a prisoner to sugar and flour. Not being able to say no to something as childish as a cookie really concerned me. Knowing that sugar was as addictive as alcohol was a key in giving it up.

The motivation to stay on this change journey is very spiritual for me and yet it started and continues by physical acts of what I eat and how I move, fueled by my mind, will and emotions. In other words, it involves my total being. All of me has to be on board with this or I will fail.

ACTING INTO CHANGE

I can't spiritualize myself into change, nor can I think or feel myself into it. I must act myself into it because I know the spiritual, emotional and intellectual reasons behind it. I must commit. Starting the journey was definitely the hardest part. Once I started, though, there was no turning back. There was and is such freedom in walking the journey I know God wants me to walk. If my foot strays off the path in this direction or that, He points me to the right way.[5] That's why this is the easiest hard journey I've ever walked. He walks beside me every step of the way. With my hand in His, how can I fail?

For me, part of walking this journey had to do with having a mentor who understood and gently challenged me to stretch myself further. That person was Russ. He is without a doubt the one who has taught me the most about the change process and God's involvement in that process. It's not magic. It takes intentional effort — one foot in front of the other, one choice at a time. In his words, "If losing weight was easy, everyone would do it."

I'm indebted to him for sharing his own change story with me. It was when I heard his story that the finger of God rested heavily on me and sent me in the direction that changed the entire trajectory of my life.

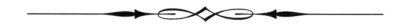

CHANGE STORY
RUSS HARDESTY

An addiction is anything I allow to control my life. In my case, it was alcohol, which related somewhat later in my life to my propensity for sugar. Before I began my change work where alcohol was concerned, I was in the process of growing my cognitive behavioral therapy counseling practice. My wife and I decided it would be helpful do a regular kind of program for those with alcohol-related challenges.

We took our team to a training session to prepare to offer an intervention program for DWI offenders. After the first evening of training, the trainer and her staff invited us to go with them to the local bar.

PERSONAL INTEGRITY

Drinking alcohol with others who were going to help still others stop drinking alcohol, triggered something in me. It seemed this behavior was incongruent or inconsistent with who I was. If I was going to be working with individuals and teaching them to deal with their alcohol dependencies through abstinence, I needed to be willing to go and do the walk.

It challenged my personal integrity because I had a harmful involvement with alcohol myself. I was not above the problem. I was in the midst of it.

In learning more about the effects of alcohol on the human body, a striking bit of information to me was that two to three drinks per week increases the probability of an early onset of cancer, heart disease, diabetes and other life-threatening situations. It didn't make sense for me to continue my relationship with alcohol from that standpoint.

Being husband and father was more important to me than alcohol.

At the time, I drank on the weekends, not so much during the week. I would often spend Saturdays with friends drinking alcohol. On Sunday afternoons, I was unavailable to my family due to being tired from recovering from the effects of alcohol. This awareness was another incentive to examine my relationship with alcohol. Being husband and father was more important to me than alcohol.

I drank, at first, out of a need to be social. From there it became habitual. I was at risk professionally and legally from driving under the influence. Financially we were struggling. The last thing I needed was to be spending money on alcohol. It controlled me rather than me controlling it.

I have a family history of cardiac problems. My grandfather died when he was 60 from a massive heart attack. Other members of my family died from heart and renal diseases. This is a weak physiological link in my genetics. I understood, given modern medicine, that if I had a stroke I would probably survive, but would become a great liability to my family, the people I cared about the most. The last thing I wanted to do was present myself as impaired, not able to contribute to the family and become an emotional and physical burden.

All of these issues culminated in a moment of change for me. On March 25, 1986, at an anniversary dinner with my wife, I took my last drink. I made the decision I would not knowingly do something to my body that would create a problem for people I care about. I wanted to be as healthy as I could for as long as I could.

I decided the people I love — my wife and children — were important enough for me to change my behavior and my relationship with alcohol. I decided that my behavior needed to be consistent with who I am. My actions needed to be consistent with my character.

A big part of that for me was thinking of the future when my children would be older. I wanted to be there. I wanted to be a part of their lives. I understood that for my children to learn to respect themselves, they needed a model of someone who respected himself, too.

> My actions need to be consistent with my character.

This was a pivotal point of personal change for me, but it was also a pivotal point for my family. Whether they realized it or not things would change for them because I, as the father and husband, made a stand and decided to get in touch with my purpose.

Once I made a commitment to be congruent with what I do and who I am, I began to grow in many ways. The awareness of myself empowered me to be more effective at work as a counselor and at home as a dad and husband. It started me on a journey of personal growth that has allowed me to experience success I never imagined could be in my life. To this day, I am keenly aware that my continued success is based on my continued commitment to abstinence from alcohol.

The old adage that one is too many and a thousand is not enough is so powerful. It also underlines the concept that 99 percent is such a burden, but 100 percent is a piece of cake.

PROCESS OF RECOVERY

Any kind of change involves passion and commitment. One of the errors of thinking I have observed in people is they believe they have to have a passion or feeling before they commit to change. This is why many people say, "I'm going to stop drinking, stop smoking, change my eating patterns, start exercising. I really want to do this."

They get all pumped up thinking they have to have all this passion for it before they can start, but passion runs out if there is not commitment. Commitment has to do with knowing the reason why.

My "why" was strong. It was for my own health, my love for my family and my children and for their well-being. Because of that I made a commitment not to use alcohol. Period.

On this journey of recovery, I needed three kinds of support — others, another and the Other. I had the good fortune of working with others who were also on this journey of being alcohol-free. I was actually leading them on their journey. I shared with them my decision and we became each other's support system. They became my others, along with other groups such as AA and also a personal growth study group.

I needed a mentor or mentors to confide in, someone other than my wife to be a partner in this journey. They needed to be someone who was farther along than I, but still a peer who would listen and understand. I call them "another." I was fortunate to have several individuals in this category.

I also desperately needed the Other or my higher power. I call my higher power, God. As my faith began to increase and grow, so did my understanding of God's grace, which allowed me to have greater compassion and acceptance of others' struggles.

My understanding of God grew tremendously. I realized He is a God of grace and acceptance rather than a rule and record keeper. Because of His grace, I began to experience greater freedom from guilt and shame.

ANOTHER TYPE OF RECOVERY

Wonderful things were happening in my family, my counseling practice and Freedom Seminar, a personal growth seminar we had started, but then I went to the doctor for some shortness of breath.

I wound up in the hospital having a five-way heart bypass. My main artery was 100 percent blocked and the other four were 85 to 90 percent blocked. That was 12 years ago, 16 years after giving up alcohol. I was the same age my grandfather was when he died from a heart attack.

My cholesterol was in normal limits, but the triglycerides were off the chart. This is in direct relationship to carbs, particularly sugars. Alcohol is essentially liquid sugar. I hadn't been drinking alcohol, but I continued to indulge heavily in sweets — pies, ice cream, cakes, pastas. My heightened triglycerides were in response to that. We don't hear much about triglycerides, but they are killers.

I had observed that when individuals ceased using alcohol, their intake of sodas, such as those with lots of sugar and high caffeine content, increased tremendously, as well as eating giant chocolate candy bars with peanuts and caramel. Then, I began to understand more closely the connection between alcohol and sugar.

> I began to understand more closely the connection between alcohol and sugar.

Sugar has an addictive quality to it. For instance, every afternoon I would get this sense of being flat and kind of drowsy, so I'd eat a candy bar or something sweet about 3 pm. It felt like it did something for me cognitively to help my brain function for a short period of time.

This can be very addictive. With sugar, I could actually feel the sugar high. I knew when I had a big dose. I don't have those concentrated amounts of processed sugar any more.

After my open-heart surgery, my eating habits changed tremendously. I realized the same thing regarding the possibility of being a burden on my family could happen if I continued to eat processed sugars whenever I pleased.

These days, I rarely eat sweets. When I do it's in the form of honey. We have honeybees, so we only consume our own raw honey. I drastically cut back my carb intake. I am mindful of how much bread I eat. I rarely eat pasta.

We raise almost all of our foods, vegetables and a lot of our fruit and preserve by freezing. We raise our own potatoes, sweet potatoes, winter squash-type plants, dry and green beans. We also have cattle. Much of our meat is farm-raised, mostly grass-fed with some corn products. Everything is organic, with no pesticides. We know it is healthier for us and our extended family and friends.

Good food is a building block of life. It helps us be and do what we were put here on earth to be and do. It is so easy to allow various foods, especially carbs, to dictate how and what we eat if we give control over to what we crave.

> Good food helps us be and do what we were put here on earth to be and do.

Taking back control for me means to be moderate in what I eat. I'm mindful of the source of the food. I'm mindful of how much salt I use. I'm mindful of how it makes my body feel. I'm mindful of what I need to fuel my body.

Even though we had a garden before, we really began to focus on raising our own food and bees after my surgery. My wife has a degree in horticulture and I'm a farm boy from way back. We love working in our gardens, which are over an acre. By the way, she has her garden and I have mine.

In this process, I lost about 30 pounds. My pivotal moments weren't just about alcohol or weight loss. They were about focusing on abundant life and healthy living.

FUTURE

I take things one day at a time. I know the addictions I have are with me for the rest of my earthly existence. How I live today continues to be a daily decision. I am mindful I have a pattern where alcohol and sugar are concerned. I'm also aware that if I am around alcohol today, it is easier for me to not use than it was 28 years ago. I am also aware that I cannot use alcohol in the future, but it is still a daily choice.

There are times I think, well one drink wouldn't be too bad — one drink wouldn't hurt a lot. However, I go back to the idea that commitment precedes passion. Abstinence from alcohol is a commitment I made. I am often in professional meetings where alcohol is served. I continue to make that decision in every situation.

For me to have a belief that I will never drink again or that I have arrived would be the beginning of me standing on a slippery slope. I am arriving, but I have not arrived at that place. I will be arriving until I finish this life.

It would not be worth ruining the life I have created for a moment of personal pleasure, which a drink of alcohol or downing a huge candy bar might bring. The metaphor I have for it is simple. I have a really large saving account I am creating each day, but I only get one withdrawal and I start all over again. Any withdrawal takes it all out. It is similar to the story of Esau.[6] He took one withdrawal and lost the whole thing for a pot of beans. I choose not to lose my life for a moment of pleasure whether it be large amounts of processed sugar or a drink of alcohol.

My family is worth more than that.

I am worth more than that.

Russ Hardesty is a husband, father of seven, grandfather and great-grandfather of a small tribe. He is a cognitive behavioral counselor, Ph.D., LPC, with over 40 years of service helping individuals live more fulfilled lives. He gets enjoyment out of inventing new ways of doing things, farming, gardening, raising honeybees and evoking others to grow toward their potential. He and his wife, Pat, live in Hatton, MO.

ENDNOTES

1. Deuteronomy 30:19-20 NLT
2. Jeremiah 29:11 NLT
3. Romans 12:1-2 AMP
4. Matthew 16:24-27 NIV
5. Isaiah 30:21 AMP
6. Gensis 25:24 NIV
7. Matthew 17:20 NIV
8. Deuteronomy 30:19-20 NLT

CHAPTER 3

LEADING A HERD OF ELEPHANTS

W hen there's an elephant in the room, it's pretty difficult to ignore or get rid of it. It's especially hard if it's a herd of elephants. I know that because a bunch followed me around for years. Recently a woman asked me, "What brought you to the place of making real changes to get free of the elephant in the room?"

The idea of the elephant in the room is an interesting one. To whom or to what does the elephant refer? Is it just one elephant or many? When we answer those questions, we may be able to get at the truth. So let's go on an elephant hunt.

I AM THE ELEPHANT

We have met the elephant and she is us. If we are overweight or obese and beyond, we think the elephant refers to us. I sure did.

Every Sunday when I walked in the door of my church, I would automatically look around to see if I was the largest person in the room. If I was, I would cower as far back as I could. I didn't want my elephant size to be too overwhelming.

I truly hated being the largest person in the room. If there was even one person I deemed larger than me, I'd breathe a sigh of relief. Since losing weight I know that most folks don't mentally calculate the weights of all those they encounter. Most are too busy calculating their own shortcomings to notice anyone else's.

Size is irrelevant to most. It's definitely more noticeable to those who have weight issues than others. We are the ones who have to live with ourselves. We know the difficulties our size brings.

If anything I find people are more considerate than accusatory. They are concerned for our health. They would genuinely like to help, but are afraid to offer for fear of making us angry.

SHE IS THE ELEPHANT

Someone else is the elephant. Someone made us angry, hurt our feelings, abused us, gossiped about us, hurt us physically, snubbed us, told lies about us, molested us, tried to kill us, divorced us, left us with the bills, fed us unhealthy food, fired us, threw us out, screamed at us, manipulated us, didn't love us.

There could be any number of reasons we blame someone else for our weight gain. What they did seems like a difficulty that looms so large we cannot see around it nor can we get through it. So we stay stuck and we eat.

The reasons we turn to food can be many. The truth is everyone has difficulties, but not everyone chooses to go to food to solve their problems. This elephant remains in the room because we choose to keep it there. We feed it by rehearsing our victim status. It's easier to be a victim than a victor. It's easier to blame our pet elephant than ourselves.

FOOD IS THE ELEPHANT

An elephant eats a lot of food. The amounts vary from 150 to 770 pounds a day. The larger amount of food is for elephants in the wild. They, of course, have to hunt for their own food, roam larger spans of area, endure the difficulties of temperature and terrain.

If an elephant eats too much or too little food one of several things might be happening. They don't need to consume so much food because of the environment. They can't find food or the right types of food aren't fed to them. They are sick.

All three things also affect us. Our environment dictates much of how we eat. If we are in an area that doesn't have access to highly processed foods, we will eat less. If we have the wrong types of foods we will eat more. If we are sick or metabolically broken, we will eat more.

A person who is metabolically broken can't control the amounts of foods they eat, such as sugar, flour, highly processed foods and fast foods. They overindulge because their bodies are addicted to these types of foods. Unfortunately, these foods comprise most of what has become known as the American diet.

Ingesting large amounts of these kinds of foods has contributed to causing the craving mechanism in our brain to be messed up or broken. It recognizes something high in sugar content or an item that will eventually turn into sugar. Once it hits the blood stream it turns on the craving mechanism for more. Once the desire for more hits there is a desire for even more. Satiation is never reached.

EMOTIONS ARE THE ELEPHANT

Emotions can loom larger than an elephant in our lives. They invade the secret places where no one else is allowed to go. They take over our minds, wills and behaviors. They make us do exactly what we don't want to do. We can try to reason with our emotions. We can try to force them to be silent. We can will them to be silent, but they just scream all the louder.

Paul had something to say about this. "I don't really understand myself, for I want to do what is right, but I don't do it. Instead, I do what I hate ... I want to do what is right, but I can't. I want to do what is good, but I don't. I don't want to do what is wrong, but I do it anyway ... Oh, what a miserable person I am! Who will free me from this life dominated by death?"[1]

Our emotions become the backdrop of our lives. Everything runs according to how we feel and yet, we're not really sure where those feelings come from.

GOD IS THE ELEPHANT

Sometimes we even blame God for our problem. We cry out to Him to fix us. We tell Him to make us not so hungry, to help us magically lose 100 pounds, to strike vengeance on those who wronged us. We feel if He would just do these things everything would be fine.

It's His fault for making us this way. He needs to fix us. Then, all will be well with the world. We could continue eating the foods we love and be healthy if only God wasn't so stubborn.

THE HERD IS THE ELEPHANT

In essence it feels as if we have not one elephant in our room, but a whole herd. That brings us to the crux of the matter. The elephant in the room is really a complex set of issues that involve our physical body, our physical environment, our reactions to situations and people, our emotions and our spiritual lives.

When we understand how complex we are and how we are now elephant size, we begin to believe there is no simple solution. We have eaten ourselves into a conundrum, an intricate and difficult problem.

We want to do good. We want to lose weight. We want to live and be healthy. We just can't figure out the answer. We keep trying to get rid of the herd of elephants that seems to eat what is the equivalent of their weight.

We have eaten ourselves into a conundrum.

I tried pushing the elephants out of my life. It is impossible to push elephants. They don't budge. In order to solve the problem I had to embrace my elephants. I had to own the herd that is me. Yes, I am the problem. Yes, others have wronged me. Yes, food is an issue for me. Yes, I am an emotional mess. Yes, I'm mad at God.

Admitting each one freed me to focus on the first step. For me, ownership of my issue meant I was using the key God had shown me for years. Which was that if I wanted to live, I had to take responsibility. I stopped looking for easy fixes and owned the fact that I needed to change in a major way.

LEADING THE HERD OF ELEPHANTS

Then, I turned to one of the elephants and decided to once and for all make Him leader of my herd. I realized the One I blamed for not fixing me and making me like this was the only One who could lead me to become whole, healthy and happy.

I surrendered to the One who said to me, "My grace is sufficient for you, for My power is made perfect in your weakness."[2] I asked Him to lead me to the next right step and then the next and the next and the next.

I realized it was by His grace, which is and always has been sufficient, that I was alive to make this decision. Sufficient means "enough to meet the needs of a situation or a proposed end." God being enough meant I needed nothing more and so I surrendered to Him.

My herd of elephants is corralled and led by my Creator God. There is little struggle now because I am finally Spirit-led.

If anyone can lead this herd of elephants, it's definitely Him.

I first met Rhonda Burrows when she joined Sweet Change Weight Loss Coaching and Accountability Group. She is a breath of fresh air because she gets this journey. She knows what it's like to have a herd of elephants parading through her life and she knows what it's like to give the leadership over to the Holy Spirit.

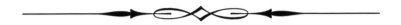

CHANGE STORY
RHONDA BURROWS

When I came home from school, Mom had baked a wonderful chocolate meringue pie. She allowed me to have a piece and I was in heaven. All I could think of was I couldn't wait to have another piece for dessert after supper. After a dinner that evening of chicken and dumplings, she would not let me have a second piece of that wonderful pie.

I was angry, frustrated and desperate. How dare she not let me have another piece of pie. I packed my little suitcase, making sure to include my 86 cents, donned my plaid coat and ran away from home. I was only eight, but even today I remember sneaking by the

The craving for that chocolate pie was strong.

windows so my mother would not see me. I don't remember where I went or how long I was gone (not long I'm sure) but I sure remember being denied that sugary treat.

Mom had explained I had already had my piece of pie for the day, but I didn't realize there was a daily limit for chocolate pie. I wasn't hungry, but the craving for that chocolate pie was very strong. It was not the only time I ran away from home, but it is the clearest memory because of the reason — chocolate pie.

Was it because of genetics that I craved sugar or was it because at times it felt like food was my only friend and companion? Was it because it helped me escape from a chaotic childhood filled with sexual abuse, alcoholic parents and tormenting fears? Was it because my mother and grandmothers nurtured me with food in the best way they knew how?

I used food to nurture myself in a family with two functional alcoholic parents.

Was it because the added weight served as a protection from unwanted sexual advances and my own sexual struggles within? Was it because the enemy of my soul found a way to keep me tied to him? The answer to all my questions is yes, although it has taken years to sort through all of those questions and the quest continues.

Food was one of the survival mechanisms I learned to use to nurture myself in a family with two functional alcoholic parents. By functional I mean they reserved their drinking for the most part until after 5 pm. Still, at times our home resembled a war zone of fighting, screaming and even some physical altercations between my parents.

On the outside we appeared to be an affluent family, but I knew I was different and no one would understand. My only sibling was eight years older than me and was a virtual recluse who escaped through reading and being very quiet. My father was also an atheist who ranted and raved against the church, so there was no spiritual training from my parents and very little gleaned on my own.

Food became my very best friend at an early age. Treats like candy, cakes, ice cream and pie were the bright spots of my life. As I began to gain weight by about age nine, I failed to make the connection between extra food and the changes in my body. I hated how I looked as a chubby child, but to give up the treats was unthinkable. They had become necessary for my survival.

ALCOHOL ADDICTION

Along with food, I discovered alcohol at an early age and then drugs later on. These only served to blot out reality, but with ever more painful consequences. God began my deliverance from all of these issues in October 1983 when He led me to a way out of alcoholism and drug addiction and into a relationship with Himself.

Previous to that, in 1979 I joined a well-known national weight loss organization for the first time. I was successful and lost 40 pounds in about a year. The difficulty came with the organization's permission to drink a small amount of light beer or wine. This turned into drinking a lot of my meals and landed me in the hospital with acute pancreatitis.

It was in the hospital that I reached my goal weight for the first time. By the time I attended my next weight loss meeting I had gained a few pounds and never actually received recognition of achieving the goal.

Over the next 35 years I became a professional dieter. I yo-yoed up and down, but increasingly up. There are very few diets, pills or plans I missed in the process with varying degrees of success, but all with the same ultimate end. When I stopped, the weight returned plus more.

For most of those years I restricted "real" sugar and used artificial sweeteners, including years of addiction to diet colas. Whenever I would start with small amounts of sugar, I would end up with binges of days or weeks of ingesting increasing amounts until I would crash and start over.

Regardless of what I ate or didn't eat, my feelings about myself were horrible. I berated and bashed myself for being fat. Every bite I took was a measure of who I was, good or bad.

I remember my late husband, Ronnie, telling me one time that he knew if anything ever happened to him, I would lose the added weight. It was almost a prophetic statement because he passed away suddenly in 2005 at the age of 50. After my period of mourning, which included a loss of appetite for the first time in my life, I decided it was time to "get in shape" if I were to have a new love in my life.

My feelings about myself were horrible.

I had a clear goal, with a stringent plan. I worked the plan vigorously. The plan was no sugar, very low carbohydrates, no salt, lean meats and mostly salads. I also exercised daily on my stationery bike for 45 minutes to an hour. By the time I met my current husband four months later, I had lost 35 to 40 pounds.

Of course, as soon as we got married and I started cooking for us and enjoying all the "good" things again, I put weight on both of us. I almost felt I should have had him sign a disclaimer about false advertising. He did not know what he was really getting.

Through many ups and downs, losses and changes in my life, my struggle with obesity remained. God began revealing things to me such as when I fasted and gave up the sugar, I felt closer to Him and I became more spiritually alive.

My denial though was that He was drawing me to more than just brief periods of abstinence from sugar. That denial helped me all the way up to a weight of 198 pounds, pushing ever closer to that dreaded 200-pound mark. That number may not sound huge for some, however I am under five feet tall, so it placed me in the morbidly obese category.

MY DREAM

I had, and still have, a dream of helping others be all they can be in God. In that process, God placed a super morbidly obese man at our church. What's more, God filled me with compassion for him instead of the contempt I previously felt for other overweight people who represented all that I was.

I wanted to help him, but I realized I could not lead someone where I had not gone. God showed me this clearly through His Word. "But I discipline my body and bring it into subjection, lest, when I have preached to others, I myself should become disqualified."[3] I cannot help others overcome what I need to overcome myself, I cried out to God.

It was in that time-frame I saw an article about Teresa's memoir, *Sweet Grace*. It spoke to me. I ordered the book and the *Sweet Grace Study Guide*. In the meantime, through her website I discovered there was a support group called Sweet

Change Weight Loss Coaching and Accountability Group. I understood the need for support and accountability after years of attending AA meetings, but this was the first weight loss support group I had found that incorporated the Biblical and spiritual principles I knew I needed for success.

I AM A SUGAR ADDICT

My moment of truth happened when I began reading the book and came across these words "sugar is one molecule away from alcohol." When I heard that, the missing pieces of my puzzle began coming together in my heart. I understood at that instant a major truth: I am a sugar addict.

I remembered back in the mid to late 1980s God told me to quit eating sugar and flour. I also knew in my heart of hearts I could do it with God's help. It became an instant commitment for me just like my commitment to not drink alcohol.

God in His loving kindness had answered the prayer I had prayed for years to give me the same understanding and deliverance He had given me regarding alcohol and drug addiction.

Just as I work out my own salvation with fear and trembling,[4] I am working out my deliverance from food addiction by the sweet grace of God and the help and support of others. I need others for accountability and also to share this miracle God has brought forth in my life.

The goal is to be healthy in body, soul and spirit. When I am caught in the cycle of addiction there are many forces at play. My adult rebellion is the same as the rebellion of that eight-year-old girl in the plaid coat with a little suitcase and 86 cents running away in rebellion.

There is temptation from the enemy to eat sugar and flour and ruin my health. Then, when I do fall into temptation, he adds condemnation to make me feel like a total failure.

Attempts to nurture myself with food came out of a misguided sense that food represented the love and comfort I always craved. Instead I've learned the true source of love and comfort is God. There is a real physical craving when any sugar or processed carbohydrates are ingested. It is real, just like the craving for alcohol was.

Another thing God has made me aware of is that for me overeating is a sin. My body is a temple of the Holy Spirit.[5] It was bought at a high price. It is no longer mine, but belongs to God. I was living in a spiritual fog because of the way I ate. The food became my god, an idol. Once I realized that, I went through the process of admission and forgiveness. Then, I became free indeed by the blood of Jesus.

CHANGES

My accountability is not only to my coach and my group, but to my God. This is also a facet of the purpose God has placed on my heart. Many Christians have been deceived into thinking eating whatever we want is okay. God has revealed to me the damage I was doing to my body, the temple of the Holy Spirit. I want share the way out of food addiction with the Body of Christ. I want to be a light God can shine through to show this can be done with His help.

The goal is not to step on the scales and see a certain number or fit in a certain size clothes. The goal is to be set free from the bondage and the struggle. This is what God is doing for me. Just as He did with alcohol and drugs, I do not have to struggle daily as long as I am faithful to my commitment to not eat sugar and the other things He has revealed to me not to eat.

I have a "three-second rule" of not looking at things I used to eat. If I avert my eyes, those foods do not get a foothold in my mind and become an obsession. I have learned to replace the things I stopped with healthy things like exercise, quiet time with God, praise and worship music and other ways to feed my soul and spirit, not my body.

I have learned ways to feed my soul and spirit.

I have been free of processed sugar and gluten for four months. The weight is coming off and I'm believing it is staying gone this time. In the process, there is major healing of my body, soul and spirit going on through the group process and coaching in Sweet Change Weight Loss Group.

I believe God has just the right plan, tools and people in place in my life at this time for His sweet grace to deliver me from all my destructions. There is ongoing deep healing from hurts inflicted by myself and others that helped to fuel my addictions.

Ah, but there is hope — hope for a life that is victorious and free in Christ. There is hope to fulfill my calling, whatever that turns out to be. There is hope I can be a witness to others who have lost hope of ever being different.

I give all the glory, praise and honor to my Heavenly Father who never gave up on me. His grace is sufficient for His power is made perfect in my weakness.[6] There is a connection between alcohol and sugar, but I am not bound by either.

I am bound only to Christ.

Rhonda Burrows is a wife, mother of three and grandmother of seven. She is retired and raises Shetland sheep dogs as a hobby. She also loves to work in her local church where she teaches adult Sunday School. She lives in Palestine, TX.

ENDNOTES

1. Romans 7:15, 18,19, 24 NLT
2. 2 Corinthians 12:9 NIV
3. 1 Corinthians 9:27 NIV
4. Philippians 2:12 NIV
5. 1 Corinthians 6:19-20 NIV
6. 2 Corinthians 12:9 NIV

SWEET CHANGE

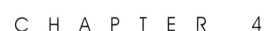

C H A P T E R 4

TRANSFORMING CHANGE

Transformation doesn't come as naturally to people as it does to the caterpillar. It was created to be a butterfly from the very beginning. It couldn't be anything else. We, of course, were created to be people with free wills. Our transformation to grace and beauty isn't as certain as that of a butterfly. We can change although it takes most of us a long time to transform.

There are many things we want to change — stop a bad habit, lose weight, quit smoking, stop looking at pornographic sites, work on that invention, go back to school. There are many ways we can transform ourselves, but many of us never start. We are waiting for a magical intervention to make it happen, but it never does. We blame God for not fixing us when all along He has given us the tools to do the job.

Change happens when we throw out the old thoughts and ideas and adopt an entirely different way of thinking and understanding. Facing the fact we have been believing lies, we put on truth. I will lose weight for my health. I will stop drinking to be a more effective father and worker. I will quit smoking because it is costly and I don't want to damage my lungs. I will stop looking at pornography because it is harmful to my mind. I will create that invention because it can help society. I will go to college and get my degree to get into the career field I want.

Change happens when we stop praying for God to give us a breakthrough and instead understand we have to stop allowing entrance to the things which now hold us prisoner. God will help us break the chains that bind us when He knows we have turned away from them and are going towards Him.

> Change happens when we stop allowing entrance to the things that now hold us prisoner.

Transforming change is something we work on with God's help. That's not a pat answer. It's just truth. It's not easy, but it will be worth it. Like all change, there is a process.

The process is really outlined in this well-known passage, which makes more sense to me in this translation. "Do not be conformed to this world, this age, fashioned after and adapted to its external, superficial customs, but be transformed, changed, by the entire renewal of your mind by its new ideals and its new attitude, so that you may prove for yourselves what is the good and acceptable and perfect will of God, even the thing which is good and acceptable and perfect in His sight for you."[1]

The ingredients necessary for change are all in this passage. Let me break them down for you in a more understandable step-by-step fashion.

Desire — First, we must have a desire to change. Change is messy business. Just ask any caterpillar trying to change into a butterfly. It's going to mean giving up some things and doing the hard stuff none of us like to do. The desire for change must be more important than staying in the comfortable cocoon to which we're accustomed.

Separation — If we are going to transform, we will be different. This means we must separate from the things others want us to do. If we want to lose weight we can't continue to eat like we've always done and bake sweet delicacies to wow our friends. Transformation will require us to be separate, making unique choices.

Alignment — Connecting and aligning our allegiance to something or Someone greater than us is not just a good idea, it is necessary for transformation to take place. Separation from the old way of life and alignment with the new must be total or transformation will be a botched effort.

Dedication — Akin to alignment is dedication. This is deeper than alignment. It means we have pledged our lives to a greater purpose and to the One who will lead us in this process. It's a turning from the old ways and turning to a new way of living every moment of life.

Action — Up to this point, everything is preliminary preparation for transformation. Now, comes action. This is where we give up cigarettes, alcohol, pornography, gambling, extra-marital affairs, sugar or anything else we think we can never live without. We start on the journey of transformation. We begin the process of unfolding our wings.

Proof — Transformation will be more apparent to those around us than to ourselves. Proving to ourselves we have transformed will take more than looking in the mirror and seeing we have wings. It will take changing on the inside. Proof may come in a moment. We may be in a situation where we make the right choice, almost without thinking and we realize at that point that we really have changed. Or we don't make the right choice, but we think through why and with God's help learn from it. This, too, is different. We have changed. There is proof. We set a marker in this place and go back to it often.

Perfection — Changing from where we were to where we are now, doesn't mean we will be perfect, but that is our goal. When we realize the God of heaven sees us as perfect because we are exactly who we were designed to be, our transformation will be nearing completion. It will never be complete this side of the universe, but we will be ready to pursue the destiny to which God has called us. We will have become butterflies and are ready to begin flight lessons.

Lindsey Summers, 20, really is the epitome of change. Her metamorphosis experience was a little different in that it was lived out in front of her high school. She determined in her heart that with the help of God she would become a butterfly. And she certainly has.

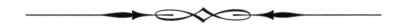

CHANGE STORY

LINDSEY SUMMERS

As a child, I was loved and constantly reminded of it. I had a family who always had my best interests at heart. Regardless of what I said or did, their love and devotion was unconditional.

Despite how often I was told I was perfect just as I was, I was overweight. Even as a child I knew this because I could never keep up with the other kids, regardless of how hard I tried.

I wasn't sporty or athletically built, so I never enjoyed gym class or recess when the other kids wanted to play active games. A few times I was bullied in school for my size and still to this day I wish I had stood up for myself.

I AM THE FAT GIRL

I couldn't buy jeans until I was in middle school because they didn't make jeans in plus-sized children's clothing. I grew up in the time where the childhood obesity epidemic had just begun. For a "chubby" girl, buying clothes which were "stylish" and "fashion-forward" wasn't an option. This brought great disappointment to me as a little girl.

The first time I lost a substantial amount of weight was when I was 10. I lost 50 pounds before the sixth grade and I felt exuberant. Finally, I could fit in with everyone else and not be "the fat girl."

However, my desire to be thin overcame my common sense. I started to starve myself. I restricted myself so much that I was only in taking in an average of 500 calories a day. I even started to lose hair because my diet was so poor.

Ten years ago I couldn't understand why my parents were so concerned about my health. I especially didn't understand when they started forcing me to eat more. They did what any loving parent would do, however, they went about keeping me healthy in all the wrong ways. By forcing me to eat more and more, I relapsed and gained back triple what I had lost. Every afternoon when I'd get home from school I'd gorge on anything I found in the pantry.

My favorite snack was spoonfuls of peanut butter with chocolate chips mixed in. I even began to stash food in my room and hide empty boxes at the bottom of the trash so no one would find out the massive amounts of food I was eating.

When I was 14, I decided I wanted to change. I joined a local group affiliated with a national well-known weight loss organization. Every Saturday morning my mom and I would go to my meeting. The first couple of weeks worked and I lost a few pounds. However, just like all of my other failed diets, I slipped back into my old ways and I started binging on food again, even the pre-packaged foods the weight loss organization sold.

> Finally, I had someone give me something to blame other than myself for my size.

By the age of 17, I weighed 242 pounds. I insisted I didn't overeat and that I ate very planned, balanced meals. My mom went with me to every doctor in town to try to get the right diagnosis for what was wrong with me.

Eventually we were sent to an endocrinologist who told me I had metabolic syndrome. He also informed me people diagnosed with this disorder typically aren't able to lose more than five percent of their overall body weight.

Finally, I had someone give me something to blame other than myself for my size, but this didn't make me feel any better.

I didn't have many friends or any social life and wasn't overly involved in any extracurricular activities. I was a recluse and I was totally content with how life was, or at least that's what I thought.

On October 15, 2011 my sister and I met with her wedding photographer to review the images he had captured on that special day. I was the maid of honor so I was in many photographs. As he flipped through the pictures, I was mortified. I couldn't believe how huge I looked. Although my "gigantic size" was mostly in my head I was still ghastly overweight.

MOMENT OF CHANGE

In those moments as we examined the pictures, I made a decision to lose weight. It was a definite moment of change. I knew deep in my gut that I wouldn't let anything stop me from losing weight this time. Maybe I was just fed up with playing victim to my size and health problems or maybe I was mature enough to finally realize the need to be healthier and live for something other than my next meal. Something clicked in my head. I fully believe this feeling of not giving up on losing weight was guided by God.

I wanted to be as pretty as the other girls at school. I wanted to look good in a dress for the prom. I wanted boys to like me. I wanted to not resent myself every time I looked in the mirror or at the scale. I wanted to stop going to the endocrinologist every three months and being told that I wouldn't be able to lose more than 20 pounds. I wanted to stop living in fear of my health. I wanted to stop making excuses for myself and be a healthy, confident young woman!

Even though some of my reasons behind losing weight were initially insignificant in the scheme of everything else, they mattered to me, as they would to any other 17-year-old girl. They were my dreams, my whys that I knew would keep me on the journey. I fully acknowledged this would necessitate a lifestyle change for the rest of my life.

The first week I only lost one pound. I was beyond devastated, I can't even describe the disappointment I felt. For the first time since I was 11, I was serious about losing weight and I wasn't seeing the results of my hard work. I swore to myself, I wouldn't slip back into my old ways. I wasn't going to let this be like all the other failed diets. This was different. This was a lifestyle change.

My eating plan consisted of restricting my calorie intake to 1,500 calories or less a day. Before this, I'm sure I was taking in well over 2,300 calories daily. This was a drastic change from my old ways. I went with the motto "If God made it, I can eat it."

> "If God made it, I can eat it."

Basically I added in foods to my plan that were more natural and cut out almost all processed foods. To this day, I still live with that saying in my head. For example, today for lunch I had a bag of steamed vegetables, yogurt, a few slices of turkey and a peach. When I was in weight loss mode, everything I ate I counted into my calorie allotment for that day. It was a lot of work and effort in the beginning, but it got easier as the weeks and months went by.

In addition, I began going to the gym to exercise five days a week for at least an hour. I began to enjoy the time and push myself harder as I lost weight. I saw the pounds come off faster as I exercised using the various machines. I still exercise three days a week for about an hour. I feel better and have more energy and stamina. In addition, I want to keep my weight at a healthy level.

CHANGES

When I began losing weight, the first thing I noticed was my face and hands thinning. Despite the fact I had lost a small amount of weight, I already began to feel more confident. I remember the first time I didn't wear a sweater over my shirt to school. I was well-known for always wearing a sweater/cardigan to cover my arms and disguise my flabby skin and stretch marks. Feeling that confident was exhilarating. That feeling alone kept me motivated.

I began to feel normal, more like the other girls at school. I even built up enough confidence to ask a boy to prom. He turned me down, but that didn't tarnish my new-found buoyancy.

My weight loss journey lasted from October 2011 through September 2012. During my yearlong mission, I discovered a new side of myself that is still a prominent piece of my personality. It's a type of confidence I can't describe.

Since I've started my life without my sole focus being what I eat, I've discovered new things that excite me. I can run up stairs three at a time. I can pick out tall boots to wear in fall and not worry about whether or not they'll zip all the way up my calf. I've discovered more of a love for the outdoors. I can enjoy summer clothing options without the need to cover my body.

> I will always have to guard myself against emotional eating.

I realize now everyone is faced with battles at one point or another in their lives. A big battle I will always have to face is my weight. I know however, I will never go back to being the size I was.

Now that I have reached my goal weight, I am still not going back to how I ate or lived. However, I am more lenient with my eating plan. I allow myself sugar, just in much smaller and more restricted amounts. This is usually at a celebration like a birthday party when I allow myself a small piece of cake. I have developed a real obsession with fruit so processed sugar is not something I crave.

The key for me is that I have learned when I'm going back into foodie mode. The other day I was at home alone and bored. I picked up a piece of fruit and ate it. Then, I went over to the pantry and grabbed a can of almonds. This is overall a healthy choice, but still is added calories. I said, "What am I doing? This is not going to happen again. It's so not worth it." So I poured a cup of flavored water and left the house to do anything, but be alone.

I know I will always have to guard myself against emotional eating. However, now I'm mindful of it and I can stop myself even when I'm sad or overly stressed. I just remember where I was and where I am now. It's not worth it to go back to where I was.

I sometimes wonder why God gave me a body that is so difficult to maintain. Throughout my life I've been jealous and envious of people who can eat whatever they want and not gain an ounce. For example, my sister has never weighed more than 110 pounds and yet ate everything I did growing up, if not more.

I resent the fact others can gorge on their favorite foods, never step foot in a gym and maintain a perfect body. However, I realize we're all faced with obstacles and challenges in our lives. My sister doesn't have problems with her weight and she'll never be considered medically obese or at high risk of being diabetic, but she does suffer with other issues, as everyone does to some extent.

I have to remind myself of the saying "God works in mysterious ways." My faith in God and His power helped me throughout my weight loss journey. God pushed me to lose weight and be healthy because He knew there was so much more in store for me besides being obese and unhappy. That didn't coincide with His plans for me.[2] My faith motivates me to never weigh 240 plus pounds again.

> God knew there was so much more in store for me than being obese and unhappy.

Now, when I browse through my sister's wedding, I take a hard look at myself in the images. I see someone who was sad and fighting a personal battle between addiction and the desire for happiness.

I also see a ghost of myself and it reminds me of how much I've grown from shedding over 100 pounds. I am no longer living as a victim of my body. With God's help, I am now a victor.

Lindsey Summers is a student at Moberly Area Community College and plans to transfer to a four-year institution in the fall of 2015. Her goal is to become a successful entrepreneur or event planner and world traveler. She enjoys being with friends and family and being involved in anything and everything she can. She lives in Columbia, MO.

ENDNOTES

1. Romans 12:2 AMP
2. Jeremiah 29:11 NIV

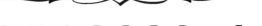

C H A P T E R   5

SET ME ON FIRE

The power of God can be an explosive fire in my life. It can if I want it to be. If I go after His kingdom with the violent zeal of a person on a mission, God promises the Kingdom of God and all power possessed therein will reside in me. However, if I allow issues such as addiction to food or other substances to control me, I will be zealous about the wrong thing. God's desire is that I have great passion, but towards the right thing.

Paul told the Roman church to "be transformed, changed, by the entire renewal of your mind, by its new ideals and its new attitude, so that you may prove for yourselves what is the good and acceptable and perfect will of God, even the thing which is good and acceptable and perfect in His sight for you."[1]

That directive alone has the power to turn lives upside down, to bring about a total upheaval of everything we've ever thought or considered. This transformation means a mindset shift in every area of our lives.

"Never lag in zeal and in earnest endeavor; be aglow and burning with the Spirit, serving the Lord,"[2] Paul continues. Zeal means to have "great energy in pursuit of a cause or objective." It is akin to what happens when a match is thrown into a forest of dry trees. Great energy springs forth with the potential to consume everything in its way.

A fire running unchecked is violent — think rampant wildfires threatening houses, cars, livestock, buildings, businesses and people. A fire with great energy and momentum is no respecter of what is in front of it. It burns everything in its path. Scripture says the Kingdom of God is within us[3] and the violent seize it by force as a precious prize.[4] It makes me think of the kind of blaze that keeps burning no matter what or who is in its way. It overtakes and burns up addictions and compulsions, which are definitely not in line with God's destiny for us.

THROWING ON THE WOOD

Jesus told the crowds "from the days of John the Baptist until the present time, the Kingdom of Heaven has endured violent assault, and violent men seize it by force as a precious prize — a share in the heavenly kingdom is sought with most ardent zeal and intense exertion."[5] Again the word "zeal" comes up and rightly so. It is an important word on this faith journey.

Jesus was telling the people that John was one who took the Kingdom of God by force. He didn't let anything get in his way. He was in prison at this juncture, soon to be beheaded for his zealous preaching. He had thousands of followers. Yet, he was a wild man living in nature. It was his strong, enthusiastic, prophetic words that people were attracted to. He knew what he believed and was not afraid to shout it from every available mountaintop.

Matthew Henry in his commentary explains that in order to come into the Kingdom, a person must "strive to enter. Self must be denied, the bent and bias, the frame and temper, of the mind must be altered; there are hard sufferings to be undergone, a force to be put upon the corrupt nature; we must run, and wrestle, and fight, and be in an agony, and all little enough to win such a prize, and to get over such opposition from without and from within."

It is far from the easy life we think it will be. It means giving up the things we want. It means facing trials and tribulations and at the same time realizing endurance is being built into us.[6] It is endurance for building the Kingdom of God.

> Entering the Kingdom of God means setting aside "the weight that so easily entangles us."

Entering the Kingdom of God is much more than attending a church, saying a prayer or walking an aisle. Entering the Kingdom is setting aside everything that gets in our way, the weight that so easily entangles us.[7] It isn't meant to be an easy journey or "to indulge and ease triflers," as Henry says.

Applying these concepts to the Kingdom of God within us is where the rubber meets the road. What is keeping us from going full-out for God? What lead weight do we carry that precludes us from running the race with the full intent of winning? If the Kingdom of God is within us, as well as around us and near us, shouldn't we be violently demolishing arguments against God and taking every thought captive to the obedience of Christ?[8]

Shouldn't we be clawing at and tearing down strongholds we've erected within ourselves? Shouldn't we be shutting every door where we have allowed a stronghold to take root in our lives? After all the Kingdom of God is supposed to reside within us just as much as around us, isn't it?

We create strongholds and we can tear them down with God's help. Strongholds are things we have allowed in our lives. Various foods can definitely become strongholds if we let them. We are sad so we reach for a sugary treat to comfort us. We are angry so we soften the anger with a piece of cake. We are overwhelmed so we drive through the fast food restaurant on the way home from work. These strongholds keep us in a daze. They make us unhealthy and unfit for Kingdom work. An out of shape Christian can't run the race[9] and be effective.

> **We create strongholds and we can tear them down with God's help.**

The zealous, on-fire people that take the Kingdom of God by force are those like John the Baptist who cast aside conventional ways, seize the moment and never let go. They approach setting up the Kingdom of God within themselves with such violent intensity that evil is repelled when it recognizes these individuals mean business. Their desire is so strong no one or no food can deter them from their mission.

The question then is this. Are we willing to grab hold with extreme force and violent intensity to make sure the Kingdom of God rules within us? Are we willing to lay aside the weight that so easily slows us down so we can run this race of faith with endurance?[10]

I know many who are willing to do just that. One such woman is Judy English. She has been a warrior for Jesus and healthy living for over 40 years.

CHANGE STORY

JUDY ENGLISH

Change is inevitable. Change can be for our good. However, sometimes we make a wrong turn or a bad decision. It might just be we believe lies in our mind about ourselves, others or our situation. Believing those lies changes us, but not for the better.

I didn't set out to gain weight, but I did. As a wife of four years and a mother to three, I felt I needed an escape. I turned to food. I gave food, especially sweets, power it was never meant to have. It became my idol.

I chose food for comfort, for pleasure, for reassurance. Eating in secret became a habit and hiding food became a skill. When my husband told me that he was concerned about my weight gain for many reasons including health, I knew he was right. I made a decision to change for myself and for my marriage.

WEIGHT LOSS LECTURER

In the late 60s, a well-known weight loss franchise came to our city. Like many, I joined and was very excited about my new adventure. Success was definitely my goal. With a motivational lecturer who was also the founder of the Missouri program and a group of friends who understood my plight, I was off and running. Our weigh-in accountability was also important. My husband was thrilled.

After losing 30 pounds, I became the first trained lecturer in my town. I also became a coach, cheerleader, counselor and mentor to members all over mid-Missouri. I cared so deeply for these hurting souls. I shared the principles of weight loss with them in each of my six weekly classes.

Success was rampant. I loved my job. Change was happening for others just as it had for me. Hundreds of pounds were gone. Outside changes were obvious. We were learning about healthy food choices, portion control by weighing and measuring food, behavior modification and preparing for special occasions. We also learned to fix food separately, if need be.

THE BIGGEST CHANGE

I realized losing weight and helping others were not the salvation for my marriage issues. Both my husband and I were weary of trying to change each other. I became desperate. I paid close attention to others who seemed to have purpose and contentment.

One friend stood out. She had marriage problems because of an alcoholic husband, but she was no longer hyperactive. She was not a flailing, angry homemaker. She was totally at peace. I was determined to learn her secret. I asked and she told me she had encountered Jesus, the One and Only. As she put it, "I am forever changed."

In January of 1972, I couldn't take it anymore. I made a decision. I fell to my knees in total desperation believing God would hear my prayer. I cried out to Him and asked Him to come into my heart and take over my life and my marriage. He heard that prayer. I was filled and flooded with love. I, too, was changed forever. I was changed from the inside out.

The desires of my heart became God's desires.[11] For four more years, I intentionally studied the scriptures in regard to food, eating, our bodies, temptation and other topics related to physical and spiritual health. I was being transformed inwardly.

As I continued to lecture for the weight loss organization, it became clear to me that inward change was needed for lasting success for all who struggle to make consistent healthy food choices. Finally, I turned to God from my idol, which was food.

Too much of any substance can be harmful.[12] Although I knew how to manage food, control portions and eat mindfully, I now began to learn how to go to God for my emotional and spiritual needs, for the aches in my soul and spirit. I was personally acquainted with the Source to help me through life's problems.

I was still lecturing. However since the organization was not Christian, I could not share my faith in a public way. I realized I could only give those who attended classes one piece of the puzzle. In my life it was so true that if change from within had not happened concerning food idols, I would have repeated my bad behaviors. For me lasting change, real daily change, comes from Jesus.

> Too much of any substance can be harmful.

I began to see people who were sitting in my classes diligently following all the food rules, differently. I understood they didn't need me, they needed Jesus. I continued to pray for members in my classes asking God to reveal the truth of His Word to them.

God's grace is more than amazing. He loves me unconditionally. He keeps on loving me. My stronghold or sin was food. He used this failure that I confessed to Him to show me how deep His love is. He used that to draw me closer to Himself.

> My stronghold or sin was food.

He began to use me to help others see their real need was a personal relationship with Jesus instead of an impersonal relationship with food. Food comforts for a moment, but it doesn't provide lasting satisfaction. Only Jesus satisfies.[13] He is the real food that satisfies my deepest needs and longings.

I resigned from lecturing for the organization. I began praying with people to help point them to Jesus Christ.[14] His death on the cross[15] made it possible for my sins to be forgiven, including the sin of gluttony and overeating. In dying, He saved me from darkness and made a way for me to live in light and have eternal life.

He began a journey of changing me to become more like Him. As I shared my journey with others, they began to experience the same freedom in Christ I had. They began to find that Jesus and Jesus alone needed to be their Source.

In the 70s I was well on my way to health and wholeness, learning how to eat healthy, exercise and feed my soul and spirit. Then, in 1981, life happened. There were situational changes, tests of faith and trials. In addition to having another child, moving twice, entering the world of work full-time and putting the ministry on the shelf at the request of my husband, we focused on parenting our four children. We were deeply involved in their activities. Life was going fast and furious as it does for many people.

I developed major health problems. I gained some weight due to medication. I experienced grief during the loss of my parents, which resulted in depression. I retired early from my career. I have since had three major surgeries including one for breast cancer.

In the midst of difficulties and struggles, I did not let the circumstances define me or cause me to lose my faith. I held tightly to God knowing He was and is the only one who is my true source and my true food. Even when things look bleak or dim, He is the Light that shines. I can never go wrong if I am following Him. Through it all, He has been faithful and loving. He loved me no matter what size I was and He longed to engage in relationship with me.

STILL, SMALL VOICE

For 42 years, I have depended on the Holy Spirit to help me with my weight control and food choices. His still, small voice points me always in the direction of food that will fuel my body. I don't always succeed, but each choice is a new beginning. I want to eat to live. I can't even remember how it felt to live to eat.

These days we have much more knowledge about food than ever before. I know how to shop the outer perimeters of a grocery store for fresh food. I have tried to focus on consistently eating some protein, fresh fruit, healthy vegetables and fiber at each meal. My husband and I avoid processed foods as much as possible. He is on this journey with me.

Staying focused while preparing meals really helps. I have learned to modify recipes. When eating out, I seldom look at a menu. If I do, I think protein and vegetables. For the most part, I have tried to be consistently free of gluten and processed sugar because I know to eat any other way will mean going back to a place I do not want to revisit.

I choose life.[16] I love freely.[17] I pray without ceasing.[18] I can honestly say that I can eat anything I want to, it's just that my "want to's" have changed. I am glad they have. I am even more grateful to my Lord and Savior, Jesus Christ, and the precious Holy Spirit who leads me, guides me. Every day He changes me and moves me always toward wholeness — body, soul and spirit. I am so thankful.

Judy English has been married for 50 years to Richard. She is a mother of four and grandmother of 12. She retired from the Leadership Academy of the Missouri Department of Elementary and Secondary Education. She loves to write, teach the Bible and do intercessory prayer. She lives in Columbia, MO.

ENDNOTES

1. Romans 12:2 AMP
2. Romans 12:11 AMP
3. Luke 17:21 AMP
4. Matthew 11:12 AMP
5. ibid.
6. James 1:2-4 NLT
7. Hebrews 12:1-2 NIV
8. 2 Corinthians 10:5 NIV
9. Hebrews 12:1 NLT
10. ibid.
11. Psalm 37:4 NIV
12. 1 Corinthians 6:12 NASB
13. Psalm 107:9 NIV
14. John 3:16 NIV
15. 1 Peter 3:18 NIV
16. Deuteronomy 30:19 NIV
17. 1 John 3:16 NIV
18. 1 Thessalonians 5:17 NASB

SWEET CHANGE

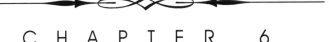

C H A P T E R   6

NO SNIVELING

No sniveling, the sign on the wall of the gym reads. I have to admit, I don't like that sign. There are times when I feel like sniveling, especially when the trainer is pushing me and I think I can't last another minute. I looked at that sign every day for almost two weeks before I went to the dictionary to see what the word really meant. I was surprised to find that the real meaning has to do with nasal mucus?

It means "to complain or whine tearfully, to run at the nose." This is good. This means maybe I can run at the mouth if I want. When my kids were growing up I had a refrigerator magnet I loved to point to, sort of an 11th commandment. It said, "Thou shalt not whine." I think the sign in the gym should be revised to say that because I don't snivel, but I sometimes whine.

IN TRAINING

Really, though, the trainer would ask for it. He would say after we'd done a set of exercises. "So how does the hamstring feel?" I'd look up at the "No sniveling" sign and say something like, "Well, it kind of hurts." And then in the nicest sort of way, he would say, "Good that's what's supposed to happen."

No, I've always thought hurting was bad. In reality, though, I'm coming to the slow realization that in order for me to get to the place where I can walk without pain, I'm going to have to strengthen lots of muscles. In order for that to happen, it is going to cause some, if not quite a bit of pain.

Although I had to stop seeing the trainer because of the expense, I have continued to do the exercises he taught me. One goal I have is to walk a 5K. Recently, as my brother says, I dipped my big toe in a 5K. I was able to walk about half the course. One day, I will walk the entire course. It is a goal I can envision. I can taste and almost touch. It is something I want badly. And, I'm willing to pay the price of training to get there.

> In order for me to walk without pain, I'm going to have to strengthen lots of muscles.

Remember the saying, "No pain, no gain?" I never liked that phrase. I never wanted to know the meaning. I'm learning it now. In actuality, I'm finding it quite empowering to feel my hamstrings and quads start to become stronger. In the past, I never really physically trained for anything or put my body "into strict training."[1] However, just as we train physically, we need to train spiritually. Those kinds of physical versus spiritual analogies never held much meaning for me.

I remember in public school having to run a mile around a track. I also remember the humiliation of not being able to even walk a mile. I remember the taunts of classmates passing me. These thoughts were going through my mind when I was on a family message chat prior to the 5K. My brother was

74

asking what finish times my cousins, nieces and nephew were shooting for. One niece said 50 minutes. My nephew, brother and cousins were at 30 minutes. Another niece had a goal of 24 minutes.

I knew I couldn't complete the race, especially in the time frame of two hours, which was when they would close the course. Maybe, though, I could walk one-fourth of the course. I felt a bit like a failure. However, I posted that I had walked a mile that day and maybe I could do part of the course.

My niece, the one who ran the course in just over 24 minutes, posted congratulations for walking a mile. It felt good to have that acknowledgement. It was an accomplishment for me to walk a mile and I knew I would try to walk a part of the 5K. I actually did walk about half of the course in about 50 minutes. As I continue to do my exercises and walk daily, I know I will one day achieve the goal of the entire course. Then, I will need a new goal.

EYE ON THE GOAL

The key is to keep my eye on the goal, the finish line, and not to be like a runner who meanders everywhere or a boxer who wastes his punches. It makes sense to me. If I never had a trainer, I might be wasting my effort on exercises that don't help me reach my final goal of being able to go the distance.

Our goal as Christians is much stronger than any physical goal. We should be like Jesus who didn't snivel or whine because of the daunting task ahead of Him.[2] He was going to die on the cross. However, He knew why. He knew the joy that was waiting for Him once He got through this valley we call life. It was worth discomfort, shame, rejection, even death, because He knew the resurrection was coming. His eye was on the prize.

It's easy for me to whine and make excuses for things I really want to do, but think I can't. My legs hurt. My foot hurts. It's cold. I don't know the course. I don't have enough time. I'm on a deadline. It's a holiday. People might laugh at how slow I walk. There's no way I can finish, so why try?

> If I stay where I've always been, I'll never go where I've always wanted to go.

If we are looking at Jesus as our role model, we will probably find all of our excuses sound like loud snorts of snivel. If there is a task God is challenging me to do, I know it is for my own good. It will take discipline, courage, even faith, but it will be worth it in the long run. It might even take me into some uncomfortable situations that cause a little pain. However, if I always stay where I've always been, I'll never go where I've always wanted to go. God knows that. That's why He prods me to venture out of my comfort zone. Not too far, but just far enough for me to get the thrill of accomplishment.

Nothing fuels motivation like success, even a small success.

That's why I challenge myself with these questions. What is the dream I have? How badly do I want it? Am I up to the task? What is my first step to reaching that goal? What will I do about it today?

No sniveling. No whining. I'm going to keep my eyes on Jesus. I'm after the prize. My brother, Mark Randall Shields, was playing the role of Jesus before the 5K. He needed two more family members to make the second team of four. He didn't push. However, he knew there was this desire inside of me to actually try. He just told me I could do it. I'm proud of my brother's weight loss and his passion for running and biking. He is one of my heroes.

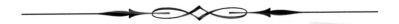

CHANGE STORY
MARK RANDALL SHIELDS

I love studying the motivation of behavior change. Seven years ago I was morbidly obese, 100 pounds over a normal BMI — an overweight, out-of-shape behavioral health counselor with 30 years of experience trying to help others change their addictive, self-destructive behaviors.

William Miller first began articulating a motivational approach to behavioral change in 1983. Motivational interviewing is a non-judgmental, non-confrontational and non-adversarial approach that attempts to increase a person's awareness of the potential problems caused, consequences experienced and risks faced as a result of problem behavior.

If motivation was a mathematical formula, it could be viewed like balance scales. When awareness of the reasons to change outweighs the reasons to stay the same, behavioral change will happen.

I believe my change was a product of moments of clarity increasing motivation and successes, increasing confidence in my ability to change.

Awareness of a problem without confidence or faith in ability to change is depressing. As a food addict I self-medicated depression with overeating. It's a very sad, lonely, depressing, deadly life.

Seven years ago I was close to 300 pounds. I desperately wanted to lose weight and be fit. So I tried every diet that came along. Nothing seemed like a permanent solution.

I remember thinking I'll lose X amount of weight and then I can be "normal" which translated to stop dieting and start eating again. Needless to say with that thinking error, I always put the weight back on and usually gained even more.

After many failures, I began to lose confidence in my ability to ever lose weight. Sometimes I would cope with the failure by convincing myself I was not that overweight. We humans really have a remarkable capacity for self-deception. However, most of the time I knew I was obese, at greater risk for early death and that my weight was interfering with my lifestyle.

> Awareness of a problem without confidence or faith in ability to change is depressing.

I figured maybe I would never be able to lose weight. Maybe I would just eat myself to death at an early age. I knew my body could not sustain the weight I was carrying for long. I had high blood pressure, high cholesterol and gout. In those dark moments I thought I was destined to die early of a weight-induced heart attack.

FINDING MOTIVATION TO CHANGE

What gave me the motivation and confidence to change? A two-year-old, an objective feedback group support, a healthy diet and exercise. These moments of clarity led to the acceptance of my obesity.

When my first grandson was born, I was able to spend a lot of time with him. As my relationship with this new life grew, so did my desire to live. At about two years of age he stuck his arm up to his elbow into my flabby midsection and told me I needed to lose my "fat belly."

I couldn't deny it. His blunt childlike honesty cut through the layers of flabby denial and focused my motivation. I started thinking about all the milestones in his life I would miss if I didn't get healthy — watching him grow up, graduate high school, become an adult and have a family of his own. I didn't want to subject my family and grandchildren to my preventable death at an early age.

> My two-year-old grandson told me I needed to lose my "fat belly."

Because of a project at work, I learned the criteria for metabolic syndrome and other risk factors associated with major health complications and premature death. I compared myself to the population that meets criteria for inclusion in a special disease management program. I realized I had the same risk factors — BMI over 30, waist circumference over 40 inches, high blood pressure and high cholesterol. It was hard to deny. I was killing myself with food.

A few years ago I was referred to a cardiologist for a stress test because of some discomfort I felt while running. I had already lost 40-50 pounds and was feeling pretty good about myself. But the cardiologist was straightforward and did not "sugarcoat" the feedback and the answers to my questions. He said it was great I was running and to keep it up. However, in order to be in a lower risk group I should lose more weight and inches around my waist. I had lost some weight, but I was not sure how much more I could lose. He answered my question with a familiar bluntness and said I should be around 200 pounds. At 250 pounds, losing another 50 with the methods I had been using seemed almost impossible. Then, he handed me a piece of paper and said following this plan would help me lose weight, drop inches around my waist and decrease cholesterol.

GAINING CONFIDENCE TO CHANGE

Seven years ago my workplace started a group weight loss competition. I agreed to be on a team not knowing if I could lose any weight, but desperate to do so. I did lose weight and my team won. In subsequent years, I participated in many more of these group weight loss competitions and learned some valuable lessons.

First, group or team support for weight loss works. Being able to chat about challenges and successes and being committed to a team helps. Second, small rewards like a couple of dollars for winning the week are surprisingly motivating. Third, public acknowledgement of success as the winning team and conversely public embarrassment of poor team performance, uncovered some useful competitive drive.

Fourth, dramatic short term weight loss caused by starvation dieting is not sustainable and a rebound weight gain always followed the end of the competition. I gained some confidence in my ability to lose weight in the short-term, but my inability to maintain the weight loss was depressing. I knew something was missing.

The piece of paper the cardiologist handed me turned my life around. The Duke Lipid Clinic Low Glycemic Index is a simple one-page document. It has three columns of food items listed labeled low, moderate and high. The instructions are simple — eat mostly food in the low glycemic index column. Occasionally you can eat from the moderate glycemic index column. Avoid eating the foods in the high glycemic index column.

My wife continued to love me and never complained about my weight.

Susan, my wife and best friend, has more to do with my recovery and weight loss than anyone. When we first met, I had been biking, lifting weights and was somewhat physically fit at about 245 pounds. Susan does not share my food addiction and seems to naturally maintain a healthy weight. As I slowly gained 50 pounds, she continued to love me and never complained about my weight. The closest she came to complaining was occasionally verbalizing her concern I might die of a heart attack. Now, she is my healthy weight and fitness cheerleader.

Every time I wanted to start a new diet she was right there, cooking and following the new diet with me. She would lose weight on whatever new diet I tried. I would lose and then gain it back. When I brought the low glycemic index diet back from the cardiologist visit, she was immediately on board and started preparing meals following the plan.

I transitioned to a new way of eating and a new way of thinking about food.

I remember being a little frustrated at first as she lost more weight than I did in the first month. The difference is she does not have a food addiction and the low glycemic index plan's high focus on vegetables and non-processed foods was closer to her normal lifestyle.

Susan has always been adventurous when it comes to food. She loves new food and new restaurants. I looked to food for comfort, not adventure. I was comfortably killing myself in my meat-potatoes-bread-dessert rut.

As a kid, I hated vegetables. I was the "picky eater" who wouldn't eat them. Surprisingly, some foods I avoided all my life I have now discovered I really like. To break out of the comfort food rut, I had to develop new attitudes and relationships with food. The universe rewards action, therefore sometimes the first step for me was trying new vegetables. Then, I set a goal of trying new low glycemic foods regularly. Eventually I transitioned to a new way of eating and a new way of thinking about food.

Following this new healthy eating plan involved eating new foods and avoiding high glycemic index foods. The foods I avoid include traditional high carb items like cookies, candy, cakes, pies, doughnuts, potatoes, French fries, pasta and white bread. However, foods I used to think were healthy like baked potatoes, whole grain bread and watermelon are also on my list to avoid.

I have been following the low glycemic healthy eating plan for two years and have been completely free of refined sugar for one year. I have to say, my sister, Teresa, was right about refined sugar. I found I am a person who can't eat just a little. I learned this the hard way when I tried to do that during Thanksgiving 2013. In order to not let it control me, I now stay away from it completely.

I finally have a healthy, more stable relationship with food. Giving up high glycemic foods decreased cravings and gave me more control over what I eat and how much I eat. I'm in recovery from a food addiction and just like other addictions I'm better off if I completely avoid the foods I am addicted to. Lucky for me, some smart people came up with a simple healthy eating plan, which helped me classify foods I should leave alone.

> I finally have a healthy more stable relationship with food.

I'm a person in recovery from an eating disorder I call a food addiction. Because I'm in recovery, I've lost over 100 pounds in the last seven years. I am finally in the normal BMI range with the lowest weight I have been in 30 years. My fitness level has improved dramatically. I don't believe running made me thin, but getting thin allowed me to run.

I now understand the phrase "you can't outrun a bad diet." I started exercising along with changing what I was eating. As I lost weight, I transitioned from walking to bike riding to weight lifting to running. Seven years ago I couldn't run 50 feet, now I run 20 miles a week and run 5K races for fun. I ran my first half marathon this summer.

> We always need to challenge ourselves with growth opportunities.

I can run and play with my seven grandchildren. I can say yes to life and adventure. I look forward to the physical challenge of a summer mountain hike in Colorado. I have enough energy to tackle home improvement projects on the weekends and evenings, something I love to do, but was having problems doing at my previous weight.

Fitness is about individual challenge and growth, about patience, sustained effort and pushing beyond your comfort zone. In a lot of ways it's a metaphor for life. We always need to challenge ourselves with growth opportunities.

As I throw the football to my grandson and run up the hill to tackle him or run down the street to the park, I am reminded that seven years ago I was a couch potato unable to run and play with the kids. I really didn't want that type of relationship with my grandchildren. I can keep up with the kids and I'm looking forward to years of fun, adventure and the legacy of grandchildren.

Recovery from food addiction, which seemed like an obstacle that couldn't be overcome, gave me new energy and confidence. Today, I'm not busy eating myself to death; I'm busy running towards life.

I Run

For fitness

For challenge

For fun

For family

For strength

For serenity

For legacy

I run for life.

Mark Randall Shields is a behavioral counselor and ATR Project Director for the Missouri Department of Mental Health. He and his wife, Susan, have six children and seven grandchildren. He enjoys running, biking, fishing, camping, hiking and Mizzou sports. He lives in Jefferson City, MO.

ENDNOTES
1. 1 Corinthians 9:25 NIV
2. Hebrews 12:1-2 NIV

SWEET CHANGE

SWEET GOLD

Something lies buried inside us. It's been there for a very long time. Actually it's been there since before we were born. It's precious, rare and pure. It's the essence of who we are and who we become when we are in Christ. It's sweet gold.

It's no accident that one of the gifts given to the baby Jesus by three supposed very wise men was gold.[1] It's also no accident that the streets of heaven are paved with pure gold, transparent as glass. Or that gold adorned the Temple of the Lord.

Gold is the most expensive and most precious metal. It is something that man cannot duplicate. Its worth is in its rarity. Because of this it represents God's divine nature — the only nature having immortality. Is it not interesting that God bestows that same eternal life on believers when they accept Jesus's sacrifice for their human sin nature? "For God so loved the world that he gave his one and only Son, that whoever believes in him shall not perish but have eternal life."[3]

This same symbol of the divine nature of God was given as a gift to Christ as a baby, as an indication of who He was. The golden streets of heaven are another indication of that divine nature.

In several places, God speaks of the process of bringing His people back to Him as refining them like gold or silver. "I will put them into the fire; I will refine them like silver and test them like gold. They will call on my name and I will answer them; I will say, 'They are my people,' and they will say, 'The Lord is our God.'"[4]

The testing or purification process takes all the impurities out of gold. In the same way, God wants the impurities removed from the lives of His people so they will be fully devoted to Him.

Peter explained it this way: "Pure gold put in the fire comes out of it proved pure; genuine faith put through this suffering comes out proved genuine. When Jesus wraps this all up, it's your faith, not your gold, that God will have on display as evidence of his victory."[5]

WISDOM'S GOLD

So what is the hidden gold inside of us? In essence, it's a total reliance on the wisdom of God and His Word for everything. It's following Him in all His ways. It's learning that everything necessary for walking life's journey in victory is found in Him.

Consider this statement from Proverbs when wondering what to do. "Wise correction is more valuable than silver or gold. The finest gold is nothing compared to the revelation-knowledge I can impart. Wisdom is so priceless it exceeds the value of any jewel. Nothing you could wish for could equal her."[6]

God wants us to tap into His resources — His gold. It is found only when we look to Him instead of to ourselves. If we are directionless, we need to go to Him and ask for directions. Otherwise, we will remain lost and without value in the Kingdom.

"If you wait at wisdom's doorway — longing to hear a word for every day, joy breaks forth within you as you listen for what I'll say. For the fountain of life pours into you every time you find Me, and this is the secret of growing in the delight and favor of the Lord."[7]

This golden walk in wisdom with the God of the universe happens when we focus on Him and His wants instead of our own fleshly desires and wants. Although we live in a body, we do not have to fulfill every whim, desire or craving we have. These can be anything related to the body — sexual sin, pornography, overeating, over-the-top anger, jealousy, theft, overindulging in alcohol or other things we think we must have to satisfy this craving that we can't seem to satisfy any other way.

> We do not have to fulfill every craving we have.

John tells us, "Don't love the world's ways. Don't love the world's goods. Love of the world squeezes out love for the Father. Practically everything that goes on in the world — wanting your own way, wanting everything for yourself, wanting to appear important — has nothing to do with the Father. It just isolates you from Him. The world and all its wanting, wanting, wanting is on the way out — but whoever does what God wants is set for eternity."[8]

As I was studying the other day, I ran across a verse in Proverbs that grabbed my attention. It is exactly what God has been doing in me on this journey I've been walking. As I get closer and closer to Him and the processed sugar becomes a thing of the past, He replaces that old desire with something 100 times greater.

What I did back then was to hand Jesus my overwhelming craving and desire for sugar. What He gave me in exchange was something I always wanted, but never knew I wanted until I began to experience it.

My soul is fed everyday from the purity, wisdom and gift of the gold He imparts to me. "When God fulfills your longings, sweetness fills your soul."[9] I exchanged processed sugar that leads to slow death for the real true sweetness of being close to the Master that leads to life eternal.

I am grateful for this addiction. It is because of my weakness that I understand more fully how very much I need God's strength. I can say with Paul, "So now I am glad to boast about my weaknesses, so that the power of Christ can work through me.[10] That's why I take pleasure in my weaknesses, and in the insults, hardships, persecutions, and troubles that I suffer for Christ. For when I am weak, then I am strong."[10]

> My addiction shows me when I am weak, then I am strong.

My weakness makes me humble. It reminds me of my posture before God. It reminds me that I am self-sufficient only in His sufficiency.[11] James says it best, "God opposes the proud, but gives grace to the humble. So humble yourselves before God. Resist the devil, and he will flee from you. Come close to God, and God will come close to you ... Let there be tears for what you have done. Let there be sorrow and deep grief. Let there be sadness instead of laughter, and gloom instead of joy. Humble yourselves before the Lord, and He will lift you up in honor."[12]

We only come close to God when we know that only He is true sweetness. Only He is true gold. When we live close to Him, His gold —the essence of who He is — cannot help but shine from us.

This is the sweet gold, the gold that only He can bring into our lives. It allows us to prosper, to have good health — body, soul and spirit.[13] Prosperity is not just physical gold, but it is the fulfillment of being close to our Master each and every day.

> Walking this journey brings us closer to Him because we know how desperately we need Him.

Walking this journey brings us closer to Him than we have ever been before because we know how desperately we need Him. And He fills our every need for sweetness with His close presence.

It is my prayer that we will be able to hand to Jesus the things we crave, the things that are pulling us headlong away from Him. As we do, He will give us something much greater. He will give us Himself completely, with more grace, favor and blessing than we could ever imagine.

This is definitely the heart cry of my friend, Pam Leverett. Even though she is well on her weight loss journey, she is also finding the sweet gold that only He can bring to her life.

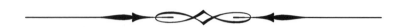

CHANGE STORY
PAM LEVERETT

S eems as though I've known what a calorie was from the time I was born — and that was 59 years ago. I never met a diet with which I wasn't personally familiar. Most of my friends didn't have a clue, but I did. How could I not?

My mom struggled with weight most of her adult life. When I was six years of age, I remember eating a delicious dinner Mom had prepared, then going with her to the rec center where she exercised hoping to burn off those unwanted pounds.

FOLLOWING MOM'S FOOTSTEPS

I am the oldest, with one sister two years younger and one seven years younger. Annie is closest to me in age and heart. We have talked for hours about family issues including habits, health, genetics and more. We believe Mom has lived a lifetime being validated by people, including us, complimenting and consuming the food she prepared. As I became a young woman, I began to follow in my mom's footsteps. I followed those footsteps to food and so began my struggle with the scale.

After enjoying some thin years, Annie eventually became my overweight sister, my cohort in food crimes. We began commiserating a few years ago and realized food was not only delicious, but it comforted us. Yes, it did for short periods. We had wonderful meals that left me wanting another helping, but there was nothing left. We tasted an occasional French twirl or cinnamon roll, but I wanted more.

When I married and left my parents' home, I became the one in control, not my mom. I could eat anything I wanted. Oreos, as many and any time I wanted them. French twirls and cinnamon rolls, whenever I wanted one or two or more. I could eat anything, and eat, I did.

In my early 20s although I was overeating, I remained physically active enough that I wasn't overweight. After giving birth to children 10 years apart when I was age 25 and then 35, I managed to diet my way back each time to what was a normal weight for my frame. After my youngest was born, I didn't bounce back as quickly. It took more work, much more dieting and much more working out.

> I became the one in control, not my mom. I could eat anything I wanted.

I had close friends who ate inordinate amounts of delicious foods and introduced me to foods I didn't know existed and sometimes couldn't pronounce — and I loved it all. My friends jogged and exercised and worked out every day. I didn't. My downward health spiral began.

I didn't believe I had time to exercise. My career as a court reporter was very stressful. I worked many hours, sometimes leaving home at midnight to visit the local 24-hour doughnut and coffee shop. My husband traveled on business at least twice a month, which left most home responsibilities to me.

I had children in different schools and activities. I was overly committed and involved at my church, not to mention taking care of my house and fulfilling God's call on me as a wife and mother. I tried to be — a perfect wife, perfect mother, perfect court reporter, perfect friend, perfect church member, perfect housekeeper and perfect cook. I needed strength to be all of those perfect people. I needed food to give me strength and to comfort me in my misery or so I reasoned.

My overeating and lack of physical activity caught up with me by the time I was 40. I was too busy to exercise, but not too busy to eat. I ate when I was under a lot of stress and I ate when I was under little stress. I ate when I was happy and I ate when I was sad or depressed. I ate when I was with friends and I ate even more when I was alone. I ate in restaurants and I ate at home. I even hid my favorite foods so that my family didn't know I was eating them or, even worse, see them and eat them before I could devour them.

It's no wonder that six years ago my doctor told me I met all but one symptom of metabolic syndrome. I was 90 pounds overweight and he added, I had to do something immediately.

BECOMING GRANDMA

My first grandchild was about to be born. Three months after his birth I was having a knee replacement. This was not the way I had dreamed I would grandparent. I wanted to be active and alive and healthy for many years so I could help shape this precious boy's life and be there when he needed me.

I knew I had to get serious about my health. I began my search for a route to lead me to health. I knew I could go back to the diet where I had been most successful. After all, as my husband said, I had followed it before and lost 40 pounds, so I could do it this time and lose 90. Could I do it again? Could I stay on the diet and get to my goal weight?

In addition to the weight gain, I had developed problems with my feet, which made a lot of physical exercise impossible. I cried out to God. I really cried out. Always before I had only asked Him to help me lose weight and stay on a diet, but after that I would attempt it in my own strength. However, I had never truly cried out in desperation.

> "When God fulfills your longing, sweetness fills your soul."

He heard my cry and led me to the book, *Sweet Grace*, by Teresa. I immediately loved the title. I mean any book with the word sweet in the title had to be for me. I subscribed to her emails. When I would read one, I would anxiously await the next. I ordered the book and the study guide. I was still crying out to God and asking for direction.

Over the next few months I reread *Sweet Grace*, worked the study guide and read the daily emails Teresa sent. I knew I was addicted to sugar. In one of Teresa's articles, a scripture moved me to tears. "When God fulfills your longings, sweetness fills your soul."[14] Oh, how I love that verse. God used it to speak to me. Could that ever be me? I wanted God to fulfill my longings. I wanted sweetness to fill my soul, but I also wanted sugar.

The turning point happened when my sisters and I sat in a hospital waiting area a couple of months later. Mom was having very serious heart and health problems. She was declining rapidly and was having a heart catheterization. The doctor's report was not good. Her heart was only functioning at 15 percent and would get worse, not better. Nothing could be done. We all cried tears of disbelief, but also tears of sadness for Mom and Dad, knowing it would never be the same for them or our family.

After a little time to adjust to the news, Annie and I talked. We knew beyond the shadow of a doubt if we didn't change our lifestyles, we would be going down the same path as Mom. My attitude began to change.

> It wasn't willpower I needed. It was His will and His power to stay the course.

Two months later I learned of the impending Sweet Change Weight Loss Coaching and Accountability Group. I emailed Teresa early on letting her know I was definitely interested in joining once it was established. I feel the book and study guide contributed to my turning point and helped me see my addiction and self-centeredness more clearly.

I will never go back to my old way of eating and living. It wasn't willpower I needed. It was His will and His power. Through the Holy Spirit revealing the path to health and His power to stay the course, I am changing. It wasn't a one-time change either. It is a constant, daily-living process.

This journey to health has not been easy. Within the first month of giving up sugar, Mom had surgery. I took a meal to my parents. One of my mom's friends had brought them an entire pound cake as a get-well token. My mom offered it to me. I told her I wasn't eating sugar and had not had any for almost a month. She said it didn't have that much sugar in it and offered it again, then began really pushing it.

I finally used a harsher tone and explained as lovingly and simply as I could that I am an addict. Just as some of her family had alcohol addictions, I was addicted to sugar and it was killing me. We had a long, long talk. She cried and I cried.Mom now supports me 100 percent on my quest to be free of sugar.

WALKING THE JOURNEY

When I began walking this journey, I came across a scripture written just for me. "A prudent person foresees the danger ahead and takes precautions; the simpleton goes blindly on and suffers the consequences."[15] I was a simpleton and I have suffered the consequences, but no more. I am now a prudent person. God allowed me to see the danger ahead if I had stayed on the path of overindulgence, gluttony and addiction.

I have been free of refined or processed sugar for over four months. Each week I set goals that involve stopping and starting. I stop or surrender an unhealthy food, action or thought and I make a choice to begin something that is good or healthy.

I have lost weight and I am moving more, but I also feel so much better physically. More than that, just being free of that which controlled me is exhilarating. As the Holy Spirit teaches me, I am learning to surrender more unhealthy foods or areas of my life.

I never want to live with anything from which Jesus has given me freedom. I never want to be identified by my problems or addictions. Just like the woman with the issue of blood in the Bible who pressed her way through to Jesus and to victory and healing,[16] so will I. If she could do it, so can I. I am pressing my way to victory.

My journey to health thus far has been an eye-opening-spirit-awakening-soul-searching-gut-wrenching trip. It has not been easy, but it's not been as difficult as I thought it would be. It's been sweet. That's the word for it — sweet. I learned years ago that obedience brings blessings.[17] I always told my children each day as they left for school "Be obedient, be blessed and be a blessing." That's my goal. I have a long way to go and I have to constantly seek the Lord, not just daily or even hourly, but constantly as I walk with Him.

> He is always waiting there to give me His hand, along with His grace and love to bring me back to that safe place.

When I was a young girl I used to play the game "Mother May I?" We couldn't move unless the "Mother" in the group said we could. My walk with the Lord is somewhat like that game. I am walking hand-in-hand with Him. He walks about one step ahead so I am actually following His leading.

As we walk, if I am having a difficult day or want to do or eat something I know I probably shouldn't, I have begun asking if it's okay with Him. I don't always listen. Sometimes I have tried to reason with Him and I admit I have slipped. Still, He is always waiting there to give me His hand, along with His grace and love to bring me back to that safe place.

He is giving me focus and strength for the journey. "Like obedient children, do not comply with the evil urges you used to follow in your ignorance, but, like the Holy One who called you, become holy yourselves in all of your conduct."[18] I always thought this an impossible quest, but now I am more aware of living in His sweet grace that makes the change of conduct possible.

Pam Leverett is a wife, mother and grandmother. She lives in Georgia and works as a court reporter. Her interests are spending time with family, gardening and decorating.

ENDNOTES

1. Matthew 2:11 NIV
2. Rev. 21:21 NIV
3. John 3:16 NLT
4. Zechariah 13:9 NIV
5. 1 Peter 1:7 MSG
6. Proverbs 8:10-11 TPT
7. Proverbs 8:34-35 TPT
8. 1 John 2:15-17 MSG
9. Proverbs 13:19 TPT
10. 2 Corinthians 12: 9b-10 NLT
11. Philippians 4:13 AMP
12. James 4:6-10 NLT
13. 3 John 2 NIV
14. Proverbs 13:19 TPT
15. Proverbs 22:3 NLT
16. Matthew 9:20-22 NIV
17. Psalm 24:3-6 NIV
18. 1 Peter 1:14 NET

SWEET CHANGE

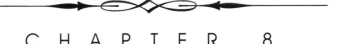

CHAPTER 8

GOD DIRECTS MOVING OBJECTS

There are many reasons to sit on the sidelines of life. Some people want their experience to be perfect. They want their home to be perfect, all nice and clean, perfectly decorated. I'll take mine almost decorated and partially clean. If that happens I will be so happy, even without my perfectionistic tendencies.

It is a known fact, however, that it won't get perfectly clean if someone doesn't clean it. And yes, I hire an awesome cleaning crew who does a top to bottom once a month, but in between the floors get dirty, dishes have to be washed and laundry put away. I can wish things were different, but that just doesn't work.

What I've learned is that God directs moving objects. I have to be doing something for Him to direct me. "Whether you turn to the right or to the left, your ears will hear a voice behind you saying, this is the way: 'walk in it.'"[1] When I get to that place where I'm just not sure of the next step, I pray for guidance and take a step. I Listen with my whole heart, soul and body for that gentle nudge from the Spirit. He never lets me go wrong.

MOVING CLOSER

Recently, God nudged me about something I was writing or wanting to write and said, "Be still and know that I am God." The word "I" was emphasized strongly. I thought it didn't fit with this motto that I'd had for a while saying God directs me when I am moving. That day, I learned stillness is moving. It's moving closer to God. That movement brings more clarity and focus than an entire month of going here and there and asking, "Is this it? Is this it?"

I came upon some road construction the other day on a road I use many times a day. As a matter of fact, I went up and down it five times that day. Each time, the trucks had moved to a different place. Just when I thought I knew where they'd be, the next time they'd moved. I figured it was just God keeping me on my toes, seeing if I was paying attention and not texting as I drive, like I had promised Oprah.

I realized this was a beautiful analogy for my life. God is directing me to move. If I am moving, things are getting accomplished. Roadwork is getting done. I'm getting my errands done. Down the way someone may be going to visit a sick friend at the very moment a doctor is discovering a cure for her illness. I would be very concerned about this world if no one was moving or only a few were moving or everyone was waiting for someone else to move.

Stillness is moving. It's moving closer to God.

Sometimes we feel stuck like we are beaten down by the cares of life. We're lying on the floor bemoaning our lot in life and don't know what to do. However, I believe God is saying, just like Switchfoot does, "I dare you to lift yourself off the floor. I dare you to move."

It's not about lying on the floor waiting for someone to discover me and help me up. It's not about forcing God to tell me something. It's about focusing on God by moving closer to Him so I can hear His directions, know His heartbeat, see where He's going and follow Him. When I lose sight of Him, it's about finding someone to help me get back on course.

WHERE TO MOVE

When I was three years old, I was playing outside with a friend. Our family car was in the shop. My dad came out of the house, patted me on the head and said he was going to walk to the garage to pick up the car.

"You play with your friend. You mother is inside. I'll be back soon."

He was a short distance down the street when my friend's mother called her inside. Without a playmate and being an impetuous sort of child, I decided to go with my dad.

I turned to see him round the corner. I started running as fast as I could. Around the corner, I caught another glimpse of him and hurried to catch up. After a while, though, I couldn't see him any longer.

Across the road, which my three-year-old mind didn't realize was a major four-lane highway, was a place with a bunch of cars outside. He was going to get the car. That must be it. I hurried across the road, went inside and asked for my daddy.

The salesman asked what my daddy's name was.

"Ernie," I said.

"We don't have an Ernie here," he said.

"Did you think your daddy was here?"

"He was going to get the car. I wanted to go with him."

"You sit right here and have a sucker. I'll see what I can find out."

I thought I was following my daddy.

In a few minutes, a police car drove up. The policeman came inside and sat down beside me. "Are you lost?" he said.

"I was following my daddy to the garage."

"I think maybe this is the wrong place. Tell you what, would you like to go for a ride in a police car? Maybe we can find your daddy."

I doubt I'd had the talk of not going anywhere with strangers. I remember standing up in the front seat of the police car and feeling important. I know that wouldn't be allowed now, but in 1956 it was fine.

He asked me my name and my mother's name. All I knew were first names, but I did know those. In a few minutes he got a call on his radio. My mother had reported me missing. He drove me home. She was in panic mode, but happy to have me home.

I thought I was following my daddy. I got a little off course. However, with the help of the right people, I got back to where

I belonged. Even though my mother was upset to find me missing, she was impressed that I had gone to a place that fixed cars and had crossed a major highway. She also applauded me for knowing hers and my father's first names.

However, she and my daddy told me never to go anywhere without telling them. My mother said I was lucky I wasn't hit on the highway. She was thankful the policeman brought me home. Her speech made quite an impression on me.

Years later, it helps me remember that just as I needed to keep a close eye on my earthly father when I was a little girl, it's even more important now for me to do the same with my heavenly Father when I'm trying to follow Him. It's way too easy to lose sight of where He's going and think I know what I'm doing on my own. Then, I wind up somewhere that looks like where I thought He was going, but I find out I'm really more lost than ever.

FOLLOWING

My journey, though, is not about being perfect. It's about following closely, listening and not being afraid to move when He says move. And as I move, it's about desiring to be directed, moving out cautiously and listening with my whole being.

If I find myself stuck, it's about getting unstuck. If I find myself defeated, it's about finding something to be victorious about. If I find myself overwhelmed, it's about finding someone else who is more overwhelmed than me and sitting beside them for a while.

It's like my friend, Aida Ingram. She found herself in a place of uncomfortable comfort and she dared herself to move.

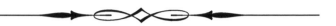

CHANGE STORY
AIDA INGRAM

My love affair with food started when I was very young. I've always loved good food, but candy was my favorite. Although I loved vegetables and ate them whenever I had the chance, candy was my first undeniable love.

It didn't start off badly. When I was young, I was fortunate enough to develop some very healthy habits, but like everyone else I also picked up more than my fair share of bad ones. Growing up we ate healthy meals. The portions were small and nutritious, all great habits when one wants to stay small and healthy.

TOO BUSY TO EAT

I was so busy being a teenager, I didn't have time to eat, but I always found time and space for candy. It was my pacifier. I thought it always made me feel better — gum, hard candy, gummies, licorice. It didn't matter. I loved them all. When I felt bad or down, those goodies always made me feel better and they were harmless, or so I thought.

If that wasn't bad enough, I picked up another really bad habit — a total dislike for water. Drinking water was like punishment, especially after having juice, a habit I still have to work hard to break. No one in my family ever made me drink water, so I didn't. I found myself drinking the calories that other people probably ate.

Back then I was one of those girls who couldn't gain a pound, not even if I wanted to. I hated being skinny. Growing up I did everything I could to gain a pound. I spent my teenage years trying to add pounds, not lose them. Not especially active, outside of doing one season of cross-country, I had my mind on other things.

Pounds became easy to put on and hard to take off.

I worked and spent my time doing more sitting than standing or moving around. It was like my body had no interest in getting any bigger. I tried everything like drinking milkshakes and eating late at night, but nothing seemed to work. If I had only known back then how fortunate I really was.

I was in my mid 20s when my daughter was born. It became very clear that not being able to gain weight was no longer a problem I would face. Pounds became easy to put on and hard to take off. I kept my baby weight and added more and more and more.

The stress of my new role of mother and wife and the emotional eating that seemed to come with it, did not help. Some of the bad habits I'd developed early came back to bite me. I drank many calories in juice. I ate candy. I fell in love with breads. I got acquainted with a plethora of fried tasty treats. The pounds came on and stayed. Before I knew it I was far bigger than I had ever been.

As a wife and a mother, convenience became my friend. High-sodium meals that were easy to prepare gave me options I celebrated and even welcomed for their convenience and ease of preparation. I had no idea those freedoms would come at such a high cost. Juice, candy, fast foods and premade meals became the formula for extra weight gain and terrible health.

My feelings of frustration, stress and worry when I was already starving for time and using food as a pacifier, only fueled my weight gain and my depression. Stressed with the responsibility of being a wife and raising a family, food became a comfortable best friend.

One day I looked up and realized I was heavier than I had ever been and I was tired. I was 180 pounds, over 30 pounds more than I weighed when I was pregnant. My health was a mess. I had high blood pressure and I just felt bad. My body was speaking and forcing me to listen. I could be of no help to myself, my family or God if I was no longer alive.

> One day I looked up and realized I was heavier than I had ever been and I was tired.

I had to change something and quickly. I realized my habits were not just bad, they were detrimental to my health and my life. My get-done quick meals were indeed fast, but they were also full of sodium and lacked real nutritional value. Doctors had a few answers, but none of them fixed how I felt. I knew this was not good.

My wakeup call was the death of my stepmom. Her death reminded me of how short life really is. It made me more aware of what I was giving up when I chose a life by default, not by design. I knew this wasn't the life I was destined to live. However, it was the life I was choosing. I couldn't blame anyone else, but myself. These were my bad choices, my bad habits and my fault. So I had a tough talk with myself. I stopped wallowing in self-pity and decided enough was enough.

I had to start somewhere and so I did. Slowly, I traded in my bad habits for better ones. Wherever I thought I could make a change, I did. Veggies and fruits were in. Sodium-filled meals were out.

> Slowly, I traded my bad habits for better ones.

Just like in that Forest Gump movie, one day I just started walking. It was an easy first step. I didn't focus on a number. I just focused on getting healthy. I started prayer walking and the walks got longer and longer. I just kept going farther and farther. Being outside and walking just seemed right. One day those walks turned into runs.

I became a mindful consumer. I found out everything I could about food and eating better. It was a real wakeup call.

I learned to stop doing things which made my journey harder than it needed to be. I asked a lot of questions. I didn't depend on others to tell me things I could find out for myself. I looked at labels. I changed where and how I shopped. I ate and tried new healthier foods. I kept an open mind. I started to treat my body like the temple[3] it has always been. Before I knew it, all of those little steps started to work.

I felt great. Every success motivated me to stay on this journey and to keep working on getting better. I ran a competitive 5K and I signed up to do a 10K. Seven months until my big goal, I was well on my way. At least that is what I thought.

Then, came the unexpected. An injury threw me a curveball. It put me at an unwanted and frustrating standstill. After all that work, a freak accident at a grocery store resulting in a bruised hip changed everything. The verdict was clear. No more running. No training. No working out in the gym. No nothing. Walking, standing, even sitting hurt. This was not part of my plan.

> Then, came the unexpected. An injury threw me a curveball. No more training.

What else could I do? Although my physical exercise came to a standstill, I still didn't give up. I could still control what I ate. I could still have a great attitude and do all I could to get well. That is exactly what I did.

For months I wasn't able to do what I had become used to, but I didn't have to give up my journey or my goal. I didn't like it, but it became a real learning experience for me. Frustrated, but resilient, I didn't stop going toward my goal of better health. I drank more water, even if I had to learn to be creative. I added lemons, limes and even cucumbers. I ate more veggies. Once I was cleared, I walked. I lifted some weights. I did what I could. Even though things weren't perfect, that wasn't a reason to quit.

It took more than six months to get totally cleared by my doctor. During that time I had gained back some of the weight I lost before my injury. I was not happy. I had to make a decision. Was I going to give up my dream of doing my 10K, or was I going to at least try?

I had 30 days to train, which was far from ideal, but train is exactly what I did. In my mind, I would rather try and fail than live with the questions. Why wonder what was possible, when I could choose to give it my all? With prayer, tenacity and persistence, I made it. Success! I didn't finish in first place and I didn't finish in record time, but I celebrated finishing my first 10K. It felt great!

As I look back, I realize that race was just a symbol of what is possible for me every day of my life. I will have setbacks. I will be frustrated, but if I set my mind on the goal and don't quit, I can still finish my race, in my time.

Even though, I am down 22 pounds, I am not finished with this journey. I will be on it until the day I die. The reality is that every day I have to choose to be healthy. It is a battle.

There will always be new and different obstacles, but there will also be rewards, like living a life I can be proud of, being an example for those who will come after me and trusting God to show me it really can be done. Every day I decide to fight, I win, and that makes it worth it to keep running the race.[4]

> There will always be new and different obstacles, but there will also be rewards.

At the end of the day our weight was never about pounds, it was and is about trust, surrender and control. The food becomes something outside of me that I believe will save me, shelter me and protect me, but it can't. It was my own attempt to "fix it," and in reality only God can do those things. Ultimately I win when I put my complete and total trust in Him, believing both that He can, He wants to and He will just because He loves me, because He does.

"Let us not become weary in doing good, for at the proper time we will reap a harvest if we do not give up."[5]

Aida Ingram is a wife, mother, minister, writer, coach and the Founder of Girlfriends With Goals, a community to empower, encourage and educate women. She loves God, learning new things, technology, travel and helping people reach their God-given purpose. Vist her website at http://www.girlfriends withgoals.com. She lives in Philadelphia, PA.

ENDNOTES

1. Isaiah 30:21 NIV
2. Ephesians 3:19-20 NLT
3. 1 Corinthians 6:19-20 NIV
4. Hebrews 12:1-2 NLT
5. Galatians 6:9 NIV

UNCOMFORTABLE COMFORT

I choose things for comfort. I love my comfortable chair, comfortable shoes, comfortable jeans and tops, comfortable height for my keyboard, comfortable-size screen, comfortable counter height — the list is endless.

Comfort's not a bad thing. We love to make our homes comfortable and inviting. When we come home we want our surroundings to be the right temperature, no annoying music playing, no loud voices. The difficulty comes when the things we go to for comfort become things we need to survive, things we would sell our first-born to get, things we must have despite damage to our health.

Some of these seem innocuous at first. A pan of brownies is not bad unless we have to have an entire batch in the morning and another in the evening just to make it through the day.

If things we go to for comfort limit our lives, they cease to be comforting and begin to make our lives extremely uncomfortable. The problem is, we've made them so much a part of our lives we can't see ourselves without them. Who are we without the extra pounds on our bodies? They have become who we are.

Why do we seek out items that comfort us and give the type of identity we really don't want? Most of the time we do it to keep ourselves from feeling something we don't know how to feel. Here are a few examples.

Fear — There are many things we are afraid of and foods, especially those made with processed sugar and bread, give us a false sense of calm. It may be fear of being alone, fear of embarking on a new vocation, fear of being asked to do something that will embarrass us. So we eat and for a moment, the fear subsides.

> Foods give a false sense of calm.

Anger — Anger is an emotion no one wants to feel. Yet, everyone feels angry at some time. Instead of examining why we are angry and processing our feelings, we tend to stuff them with "comfort" foods and all of a sudden, we are not angry. The problem with stuffing our feelings is we build a kind of iceberg effect where the world sees what's on the surface, but underneath is something that can be very dangerous.

Sadness — Life cannot always be a bed of roses. There are going to be some sad times. Most people don't like to feel the sadness and so they find some way to make themselves happy. They seek some way to at least think they are happy and hide the fact they are sad. Sadness is an acceptable feeling. Tears wash the soul. Go ahead and cry. It helps comfort much better than eating something we will regret later.

Loneliness — At some point, everyone is lonely. We can be in a house full of people and feel lonely or we can be by ourselves and feel fine. One does not always have to have someone nearby to feel fulfilled. Sugar is not our friend, though.

Eating ourselves to oblivion does not help make friends. It can actually drive friends away. Acknowledging our need at times to be with people is important. We can be a friend to someone more lonely than we are. Before long we can't remember what being lonely felt like.

Pain — Many people want to be comforted if they feel pain of any kind, emotional, physical, even spiritual pain. If there is no one around to give them the feedback they want, they will feed on whatever they can find. However, doing this can make the pain worse instead of better. If there is legitimate pain, find a health practitioner who can help. Don't try to self-medicate with food.

Control — It seems backwards to think that those who want to feel in control would be out of control with eating foods to bring comfort. However, in a strange way, eating whatever a person wants makes them feel they are in control. In other words, we are adults and we can eat whatever we want and no one is going to tell us not to. It might be the only thing we can control in our lives. In that way it brings us some measure of comfort. Obviously, it is flawed thinking.

> We can be a friend to someone more lonely than we are.

Tiredness — Those who binge and give into sugar cravings, are, of course, tired. It goes with the territory. Items made with sugar and flour make us feel tired the more we eat them. Many times we eat these thinking they will give us energy. They do, for half a minute, and then our bodies hit bottom, become

115

extremely lethargic and want more. So we start the cycle all over again.

Happiness — This emotion seems contradictory to all of the others, but in reality when we want to be happy, to reward ourselves, to celebrate, we normally go to something comforting, such as food. Even if there is no one to celebrate with, food will do the trick. It may give us a false sense of celebration, but in actuality it makes us feel worse.

Besides food as a source of comfort, there are many other false comforts we go to: drugs, alcohol, cigarettes, gambling, pornography, illicit sex, overworking, over-spending, over-shopping, hoarding and many others. Although we know the Holy Spirit should be our source of comfort we choose things we can see, hear, feel, touch, smell or taste.

We can do whatever we want, but at what cost? Paul said it best when he pointed out, "All things are lawful for me, but not all things are profitable. All things are lawful for me but I will not be mastered by anything."[1] We are free to do anything that doesn't harm another person, but what if the ones being harmed are ourselves? What if the seemingly harmless way we are comforting ourselves leads to our demise — emotionally, physically or spiritually?

THE COMFORTER

There is, of course, only one true Comforter and that's the Holy Spirit.[2] He has a way of holding us, embracing us, securing us, loving us, fighting for us and going before us to make a way. The problem is, we usually don't choose Him first.

David, one of the greatest kings of all times, knew the secret of going to God for comfort even when an entire nation was counting on him. He said, "Lord, my heart is not proud my eyes are not haughty. I don't concern myself with matters too great or too awesome for me to grasp. Instead, I have calmed and quieted myself, like a weaned child who no longer cries for its mother's milk. Yes, like a weaned child is my soul within me. O Israel, put your hope in the Lord — now and always."[3]

> The Holy Spirit is a gentleman and will not force Himself into our lives.

Jesus emphasized the importance of the role of the Holy Spirit as the Comforter, Advocate, Friend, Guide, Teacher of truth and Source of abundant life here on earth. His role is to help us in all things so that we can be God's hands and feet here on earth.

It is His sincere desire that we process our emotions and go forward accepting His prescription for comfort. The Holy Spirit is a gentleman who will not force Himself into our lives. He will however, make a way if we let Him. Begin by not trying to fix every emotion we feel with ice cream and cake. Why not get comfortable with the Holy Spirit instead? Try talking to Him. He's always listening.

My friend, Sundi Jo Graham understands this supremely. She's lost 145 pounds just by learning how to eat, when to eat and why to eat. Along with that she's learned, there is a comfort far greater than food will ever bring.

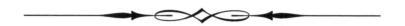

CHANGE STORY
SUNDI JO GRAHAM

There are those friends in life who aren't really friends, but they stick around like a bad cold. The friendship starts off great with a dinner and a movie and some great laughs. Then, things change. They become a curse instead of a blessing. They drag us down. They're negative. It'd be great if we could tell them, "We no longer want to be friends," but we can't. We feel stuck and unsure of what to say. Before long, they're living on our couch, using our decorative bath towels and drinking out of the milk jug.

To me, food was like that friend. It was comfort in my greatest time of need. What was meant for survival and enjoyment, turned into dependency. I tried drugs. I tried drinking. Food, though, was the one thing I could trust. Or so I thought.

WHAT FOOD DID FOR ME

Food protected me from the shame of being sexually abused as a little girl. It comforted me when I wondered if my dad would ever love me more than whiskey. It was my friend when my mom worked three jobs to support us and I desperately just wanted to hold her hand and know life was okay.

It was my friend on lonely nights when I felt like I could never fit in with the rest of the world. It comforted me as a teenager to hide the after effects of being raped. It protected me from being vulnerable with men because I feared they would all hurt me.

Food lied to me. The pizza and soda, filled with sugar and caffeine, soothed me for a few minutes when I would lock myself in my room to avoid real life. They were also the annoying friends living on my couch, using my bath towels and drinking out of the milk jug. They were not friends at all.

WHAT MORBID OBESITY DID FOR ME

In my early 20s I weighed 330 pounds. I couldn't walk up the steps without thinking I was dying. I ordered my size 30 jeans online because I couldn't find them in stores. I pretended to be happy, but truth be told, I was dying inside.

I've learned obesity doesn't just affect us — it affects those we love. At Christmas time two years prior to the start of my weight loss journey, I asked my little cousin, Caleb, what he wanted for Christmas. "I want you to ride a roller coaster with me." That broke my heart because it was physically impossible. I was determined to make that happen for him, but it didn't that year.

> I pretended to be happy, but truth be told, I was dying inside.

The next year I asked him again. His answer was the same. My decisions were devastating to this little boy. He didn't want a video game. He didn't want a new toy. He wanted to ride a roller coaster with me. I couldn't give him that. I felt so full of shame.

WHAT A FRIEND DID FOR ME

In 2008, a sweet woman named Jennifer White started mentoring me. She was an answer to prayer. I didn't yet know I was about to enter one of the most desperate seasons of my life, but God knew.

I wound up in the hospital because the stress of life had taken its toll on me physically. When I came home, I could barely hold my head up on my own. I had to move in with my parents for a month while I recovered.

> I took a short walk and came back in the house.

Then, came the day that changed things forever. While talking with Jennifer on the phone, she recommended I take a walk around the parking lot of my parents' condo. I reluctantly agreed. I'd been cooped up in a bed for way too long so I was eager to get out. I took a short walk and came back in the house. No fireworks went off. There wasn't a parade to celebrate. I didn't see it then, but life was about to shift.

The next day I walked around the parking lot again. Then, I did it the next day and the next one after that. It felt good just to get out and clear my mind. When I moved back home, I walked past the downstairs living room to do some laundry and there sat the treadmill. I had bought it brand new a couple years before. It was still pretty shiny and made a great place for hanging laundry. It even had a brand new pair of walking shoes sitting on it, which I had bought in one of my "this-is-the-diet-that-will-work" phases.

The next morning I woke up, walked downstairs, put those new shoes on, cleared off the laundry and turned the treadmill on. I was hooked from that moment on. Something about sweat made me feel productive. I had no weight loss goal. I wasn't dieting. I just knew this was the next right step for me. Each day I wanted to get up and continue taking the next right step.

WHAT LIFESTYLE CHANGE DID FOR ME

My physical habits were changing. Next in God's plan was food. I went to Jennifer's house one night for dinner and the most bizarre thing happened — she served me soup in a coffee mug. I looked at her as though she had three heads. Who does that? Is she trying to starve me to death? Where are the crackers? I knew I couldn't trust her.

In my world, one eats soup in a bowl with a pack of crackers, then goes back for seconds. The strangest thing happened, though. I was full. For someone whose crutch was food, this was a catalyst for changing the way I ate.

> The most bizarre thing happened — she served me soup in a coffee mug.

We don't know things until we're taught. I was introduced to a new way of doing things and it was life changing. The next week she introduced me to the most colorful spinach salad, full of strawberries, walnuts and chicken. I fell in love.

My grocery items quickly changed from pizza rolls to chicken, fish and a variety of soups. I wasn't starving. I wasn't dieting. I was eating to live and living hopeful for a future that didn't involve pounds of extra weight.

Before I had no concept of portion control. I ate what I wanted, when I wanted. As I've become more educated through getting healthier, I eat certain things in moderation, such as sugar, gluten and wheat. The more processed foods I eat, the worse my body feels.

In 2008, I weighed 330 pounds. Then, I went for a walk around a parking lot. Then, I walked a mile everyday. Then, I walked two miles. In 2010, I crossed the finish line at my first 5k race as friends and family cheered me on. It was awesome! Oh ... and that roller coaster ride? Caleb and I rode it twice in a row.

WHAT CHANGING MY HEART ISSUE DID FOR ME

There's a process to getting healthy. There's no quick fix that will stick. The process doesn't just involve the physical part. It involves the heart. I wasn't overweight because I had a physical problem. I was overweight because I had a heart issue. I was using food to comfort me. I was using food to avoid dealing with life. One can only survive that way for so long until the walls come crashing down and there we still are.

I had to work on my heart. I needed to forgive others and myself. I needed to work through the pain of my past. I needed to talk about my life with safe people. I needed to hear I was okay, despite my mistakes. I needed to know what God said about me and how much He loved me. I needed my heart to believe these things so I could stop using food to "heal" me.

By 2010, I had lost 145 pounds. I lost a whole person. I lost physical weight, yes, but I also lost baggage. I lost shame. I lost dependency on food to make me whole. I gained a knowing who God made me to be. I gained confidence. I found joy. Dieting became a thing of the past for me. As a matter of fact, I still refuse to use the word. I don't diet, I live healthy. If I want a pizza, I'll go eat some just not locked in my bedroom by myself.

I still struggle. I find myself having a bad day and my fleshly response is to grab food to make me feel better. I'd love to say it never happens, but it does. I'm human. Here's the thing about sweet change and God's grace, though, it's always new. If I have messed up yesterday, today is a new moment — a new chance to start over and just focus on taking the next right step.

Here's the thing about sweet change and God's grace, though, it's always new.

It's like addiction. When I go to unhealthy food, I enjoy it in the moment, but the "high" doesn't last too long before the reality of my choices set in. It is still heartbreaking to me when I choose food to fill a void versus seeking God's strength to overcome my decisions.

I couldn't be successful in my healthy living journey without the help of others. God didn't make me to experience life alone. Accountability has been key in staying on the path to a healthier me. When I'm struggling, I call a friend and we process through my feelings and emotions. I don't get it right every time, but I try. If I've overeaten, I'll call and we'll process through the why behind the what. She reminds me of grace and tomorrow being a new day.

Today, my goal is to be healthy. I've started strength training. The pounds haven't come off as quickly, but the inches certainly have. It's changed my perspective. It's not all about the scale. I'm losing inches and flexing muscles.

Each day is a new day for me — a new day to live out God's best for me, a new opportunity to focus on the next right step. I'm still not where I want to be with my weight loss, but in the words of Joyce Meyer, "Thank God I'm not where I used to be."

One. Step. At. A. Time.

My couch isn't bogged down with an unwanted friend, I'm the only one using my bath towels these days and I stopped drinking milk out of the carton, so life is good.

Here's to the next right step.

Sundi Jo Graham is a speaker, author, and blogger, inspiring others to break free from self-destructive behaviors and experience lasting transformation. Oh, and she lost 145 pounds. Connect with her on Facebook at https://www.facebook.com/sundijo and her blog at http://www.sundijo.com.

ENDNOTES

1. 1 Corinthians 6:12 NASB
2. John 14:26, NIV
3. Psalm 131:1 NLT

CHAPTER 10

CHANGING BAD HABITS

Can you stop bad habits? Can you change them? How do you start a good habit? To understand how to change habits, we need to understand a little bit about why they are formed in the first place. Many times at the first of the year we make resolutions, which are really just about stopping a bad habit or starting a good one.

According to the *Power of Habit* by Charles Duhigg, "Habits, scientists say, emerge because the brain is constantly looking for ways to save effort. Left to its own devices, the brain will try to make almost any routine into a habit, because habits allow our minds to ramp down more often."

This allows us to do some basic things over and over again without relearning them every day. Talking, walking, brushing our teeth, combing our hair, putting on our clothes, typing, riding a bicycle, driving a car and any number of activities that are fairly complicated for us to initially learn how to do take up relatively no brain power.

Our brain has stored such things in something akin to a script or shortcut used in computer programs. It saves time and energy to just hit "run script" rather than going through the process each time. The way the brain does this is through means of a habit loop that includes a cue, routine and reward. The cue and reward become intertwined until a powerful sense of anticipation and craving emerges and a habit is born.

When a habit has been formed the brain doesn't work as hard. It focuses on more difficult tasks. For the routines the brain is familiar with, the habit will take place on autopilot. Changing a habit is possible, but one must deliberately decide to replace the routine. In reality habits are always there. The brain has no way to tell the difference between which habit is bad and which is good. Therefore, no matter what the habit, anytime the cue appears, the habit loop will be activated.

Deliberately decide to replace the routine.

If we have a bad habit it's still there waiting. We can make a decision to change a habit, we can wish the habit would go away, we can will it to go away, but no matter what, it is still there.

Let's say we have a habit of eating a large cheeseburger, fries and a soda every day for lunch. It is so ingrained in us that when lunchtime comes, we automatically leave work, go through the same drive-through and order the same large cheeseburger, fries and soda.

We sit in the parking lot and eat, while enjoying being alone and putting our brains on hold from work. We started the habit for several reasons. We wanted to get alone and away from work for an hour. We wanted something filling that tasted good and would hold us until supper. Our reward was feeling full and satisfied. After having enjoyed a respite, we were ready to go back to work.

What can we do to change the habit? The cue and reward will need to stay the same. Every day at noon we will get in the car and do the same thing we've always done. To change the habit, we have to change the middle part, the routine.

We can go to the same drive-through, but change what we order. We can order a salad with grilled chicken or even a couple of grilled chicken patties without bread, along with some dipping sauce and a bottled water. We still sit in our car and enjoy the solitude and go back to work refreshed and feeling full and satisfied.

We only need to replace the routine. We may need to readjust our thinking to what we want to order, but after several days of doing this, if we have strong enough desire to change the habit, we will. From then on the brain doesn't have to think about what to order when we pull up to the drive-through. It automatically knows.

The reason this works, is the same neurological pathway that already existed has been used, but we have taken control of the routine. We can't erase that pathway completely, but we can override the outcome. The beauty of this is we can use the habit loop to work for us, rather than against us.

STOP-START

Case in point, at the beginning of my lifestyle change, I wanted to stop drinking a certain diet soda. I realized diet sodas told my brain that sugar was incoming, but didn't give my brain the high that sugar does. So then I would be craving sugar because my brain didn't get what it wanted. Thus, I bought diet sodas and candy bars to fill the craving. It had turned into a habit, but the start of the habit was always a diet soda.

There was one particular convenience store I went to almost every day as I was out and about. The feeling that I needed to purchase something because I had taken advantage of their facility was one of the culprits motivating me to buy the soda. The other culprit was giving myself a treat because I was out doing errands or my daily activities. My reward was the refreshing cold taste.

> Focus on the positive behavior that needs to begin, not the negative that needs to stop.

I decided when at a convenience store I would instead buy a bottle of artisan water, making sure it was ice cold. This worked to replace the diet soda habit. One key for me was that buying a fancier water seemed like a treat or reward to me.

This is greatly simplified, but it helps to know why just trying to stop a bad habit never works. It's very much akin to Russ's definition of stop-start. For every bad habit I want to stop, I need to start a good one.

Focusing on stopping the bad habit is definitely the wrong approach. That gives emphasis and brainpower on the bad habit. The brain, which can't tell the difference between a bad habit and a good one, will surmise this habit needs the most attention. That attention only makes us want to keep repeating the thing we want to stop. The idea of replacing a negative routine with a positive or implementing stop-start is really about an exchange. We first have to identify what the negative thing is, then identify the positive behavior to replace it with and make the exchange. Some exchanges don't seem like they go together, but in reality they do.

Take, for instance, this answer in scripture in regard to doing the things we don't want to do. "Thank God! The answer is in Jesus Christ our Lord ... So now there is no condemnation for those who belong to Christ Jesus."[1]

MAKE THE EXCHANGE

It's an exchange. We give Jesus the things we don't want to do. He gives us Himself. It's a stop-start. We stop thinking about the negative thing we don't want to do and focus on the positive things the Holy Spirit is whispering to us to do. It's a habit loop. We replace the negative routines we have always run to with the positive routines God is calling us to.

The changes we want to make can happen with some forethought into how to change the routine and what our stop-start is.

The most significant change happens when we give God the negative thing we have in our life and ask Him, "What do You give me in exchange?" Have your pen and paper handy to write down what He gives in exchange. I can guarantee, it will be life-changing.

Tom Graddy knows what it's like to exchange stress and bad eating habits for good boundaries and good eating habits. I am glad that he does because he almost didn't have a chance to experience that exchange.

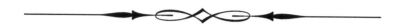

CHANGE STORY
TOM GRADDY

As a hospice chaplain, I deal with death every day, which puts a lot of stress on me. I absolutely love my job, but I didn't realize that the way I was handling stress was literally killing me.

Every person knows death is inevitable. For those I work with however, their inevitability is that a doctor has said they have six months or less to live. My job is to console the patient and the family and help them through this difficult season in their life. I love comforting people. I love being able to connect with them during these times where focus is on end-of-life issues. In reality, we all need to think about these things, but hospice patients are forced to do it sooner.

Although I tried to set good boundaries for myself and not to take on other's pain, there is still emotion involved in what I do. I cry with people. I comfort them. I talk to them in gentle tones. I believe I am fulfilling a mandate or a call on my life to love my neighbor.[2] For me there is no greater calling. Everything about me seems to fit with this line of work.

THE WAY I HANDLE STRESS

Still, there is a great deal of stress in what I do. I cope with loss on a regular basis. In the 10 years I've worked as a hospice chaplain I've done many funerals and driven thousands of miles to comfort and help our patients and their families.

I travel throughout multiple counties seeing maybe eight or more people a day. That means I'm always pushing to get to the next place and see more people. It's a crazy, hectic, high energy schedule. I was always taking care of everyone else and not myself.

On the road, the typical thing to do was stop at a convenience store or a fast food restaurant to use the facilities. Of course while there I'd buy candy bars, soda, chicken strips anything fast and easy to eat on the road. I needed comfort to get through the day and I found that in food. If I was stressed, which was all the time, I needed food to relieve my stress — sodas, snacks, treats, hamburgers and fries at a drive-through place.

I weighed 367 pounds and I had no idea what I looked like.

It felt like I needed something as a reward for working so hard. So I'd eat candy bars and soda to fill the driving time. Once I got in this cycle day after day, there seemed to be no stopping the loop.

I didn't confine my snacking and overeating to being on the road, either. I'd bring junk home, crackers and chips, and keep them under the cabinet. I had paperwork to do at home so I felt I had to eat while I did that.

A small wakeup call came when co-worker took a snapshot of me and another co-worker outside of a fast-food restaurant. When I saw the picture I thought, "Who is that? That can't be me." I looked monstrous. I weighed 367 pounds and I had no idea what I looked like.

Many in hospice work have stress-related diseases. I wasn't aware of how much it was affecting me until I injured my shoulder while trying to push a patient's car out of the mud.

I needed extensive surgery to reattach a tendon. However, the doctor said I couldn't have the surgery because my oxygen levels were too low – they were in the 80s and had to at least be in the 90s. My blood pressure was sky-high and so were my blood sugar levels. They did an ultrasound on my heart. They were scared that my heart wouldn't make it if they put me under. Going through all these tests was a huge wakeup call for me.

Time is precious. I can't waste it any longer.

They put me on medication to lower my blood pressure and on an eating plan to get my sugars down. Even then, I didn't know if I would be able to have the surgery. I had an aggressive primary care doctor who said, "Yes, I'm going to make sure you have this surgery."

Finally, I had the surgery. I lay there on the bed before it began. They were poking me with needles. I'd never been under anesthesia. I didn't know if I would wake up or not. I just thought, "Time is precious. I can't waste it any longer."

Also going through my mind was my family history. My father passed away at 31 and my sister at 40, both with aneurysms. Others in my family died of heart attacks due to their unhealthy lifestyles. Lying there I felt vulnerable. It was a surreal feeling like what if this was the end for me?

I have a wife and two children I love supremely. I want to be there for them. Nicolas is only 16 and Natalie, 18. I want to see them graduate high school, get married and have children.

As a hospice chaplain I see people every day with chronic health issues. It's not like I was never exposed to it. I guess I just never stopped long enough to understand what I was doing to myself.

I grew up as one of seven children. We ate a lot of meat and potatoes. I was heavy in grade school. In junior high and high school, I lost weight because of sports. I was healthy through college. I ran and worked out. Then, I got married and the kids came along. We were working in ministry at a church. After that, I started working as a hospice chaplain.

I realized as I lay there going over my life that I had given my medicine or help and love to everyone else. However, I was shorting myself. I wasn't giving myself medicine. With my eyes newly opened to what I was doing to myself I knew I couldn't continue to love and care for my neighbor while not caring for myself.

ON THE LOSING SIDE

After surgery, my lifestyle changed drastically. I continued with visits to the doctor and nutritionist. I followed the menu plans, which helped a lot to lower my sugar levels. I educated myself and became disciplined with the way I ate. I was focused not on a diet, but on a plan I could follow for the rest of my life.

Before this, my daughter had been diagnosed with gluten intolerance. She gets sick if she eats grains. So our family eats gluten free. I have never really been big on sugar except for candy bars on the road. I cut the soda and candy bars out immediately substituting water and nuts if I go into a convenience store.

Sometimes my wife will fix gluten-free brownies or gluten-free banana bread. Of course those have sugar, but they are not a big temptation for me. I'm not totally off all sugars, but I do watch them. I know how to work a piece into my eating plan if I want. The real triggers for me are things like chips and crackers. These just don't come into our house. It's easy because I'm usually the one who buys the groceries.

I really felt like I should do this not only for me, but that I also needed to guide our family. Day after day, I will eat a salad while they eat other things. They notice. It's making a difference in our family. Change is hard, but I know it is my responsibility as the leader to demonstrate that especially for my kids.

Nicolas and Natalie are very involved in sports. In the past I couldn't participate very much. In the last few months, I've been able to go out and workout with them. I have more energy and I'm more involved. I've been able to do this especially with Nicolas. When he'd ask in the past I'd always say I was tired. Being able to be there with him makes us both feel great.

EATING ON THE ROAD

Now, when I am on the road I bring walnuts, almonds, carrots, celery, broccoli, cheese and lunch meat without bread. Just as I used to know where I could stop to get my junk food fixes, I now know where I can go to have a good salad. I know where I can go to eat healthy.

Nine months after my surgery, I've lost 82 pounds and now weigh 285. When I got below 300 it motivated me to do even more. My levels are back down. I'm not tired all the time. I can drive and feel wide awake.

Recently, we went to a wedding and I had a hard time finding a pair of pants to wear because of losing so much weight. I have lots of pants I can no longer wear. I wasn't aware how many sizes I'd gone down. It seems like a gradual change, but it really is a huge one.

I can work my plan, which is not a diet, but a lifestyle change. Doing a diet would not work for me because I would be likely to slip. I feel like I've gotten in the groove of a lifestyle that works.

> I have things well defined as to what I know I need to live a healthy life.

This is a day-to-day thing for me. I don't have it totally licked, but I know what I have to do to live. I am no longer living to eat, but eating to live. I have things well defined as to what I know I need to live a healthy life.

I want to be around to be able to do things with my future grandchildren. If the Lord takes me home, then He does, but it won't be because I didn't do my part in regard to my health. I've been given a second chance, an opportunity to change my life. I abused myself for so long. Now, I have a shot at getting my health in order.

It's hard to be any kind of minister and be unhealthy. People appreciate seeing someone who is working hard and being healthy. People admire that. When I was closer to 400 pounds,

I did not come across the same way. I am now more believable because I care about myself.

God has played a big part in my lifestyle change. I listen to worship music, messages and the Bible while I'm in the car. I made a list of scriptures to confess. I read those and confess them as I'm riding along.

It gives me stamina for the journey to know I'm doing what God wants. I couldn't do this without relying on Him every day. I feel His pleasure in what I am doing to get my body, His temple, in order. It is what is right. I have committed the things I do to Him. I always keep that in front of me. He is sustaining me on this journey.

When I was my healthiest, I was 210 pounds. That's my goal. I'm over halfway there. I will give myself and my family this gift of life. I will continue to love my neighbor, but I will also love myself.

Tom Graddy is a husband and father of two teenagers. He is a hospice chaplain and loves gardening, fishing, sports (especially Mizzou sports), camping, grilling/BBQ and entertaining friends. He lives in Ashland, MO.

ENDNOTES

1. Romans 7:25, 8:1 NLT
2. Mark 12:31 NIV

CHAPTER 11

SURRENDER

Give Up Sugar, reads the headline on an article in the Huffington Post. It says all nutritionists agree that giving up processed sugar, not the kind in fruit, is a good idea. Because "while we all know we should eat in moderation, that can be almost impossible." Right here I need to interject a hearty, "Amen!" I've known this for years. However, it also took me years to actually surrender to it.

Corrie Pikul, the author of the article, points out that experiments show "that sugar affects the brain in the same way as morphine and other opioids do." What this means is "the more sugar we eat, the more we want," according to Nicole Avena, PhD, "and we need increasing amounts of it to keep producing the same euphoric effects."

I didn't really understand the addictive qualities of sugar when I ballooned up to 430 pounds. I would go on diets and lose weight, sometimes up to 100 pounds. As soon as I would go off the diet and reward myself with a sweet treat after being good for six months or more, I'd immediately go back into the tail-spin cycle.

For years God had given me a plan dropping processed sugar and eating less bread. I had tried that short-term and it never worked so I couldn't see how I could do it. I would sigh and try again. As I gained more and more weight and ignored what God told me, I felt more and more guilty which drove me to eat sugar and bread all the more. It was an endless treadmill from which I longed to get off.

Most people I talk to who are having a problem with weight agree with me and the nutritionists that if they could just stop eating processed sugar and flour, they would lose weight. Most, however, don't have the slightest idea how to start.

The key is in the headline and in what God told me for years — give up sugar, stop eating sugar. In other words, surrender.

Sugar is one of those substances that when I eat it, I want more. I am a person who has the metabolic makeup of a sugar addict. I can not stop eating it once I start. If I eat one cookie, I want the entire batch.

I AM A SUGAR ADDICT

The last run-in I had with sugar occurred over cookies. I consumed them because they were gluten-free, but they certainly weren't sugar-free. I had eaten five of them before I heard God's still, small voice ask me what I was doing. At the time I was eating a cookie and driving.

I answered, "I'm throwing this cookie out the window." I did and I haven't had processed sugar since. I had been eating sugar-free for several years. This slip-up, though, showed me I was still a sugar addict and always will be.

There is, however, a way to get free of sugar. And, believe it or not, it's much easier than living in bondage to it. There are essentially three phases to getting free of sugar or any addiction: acceptance, surrender and obedience.

Acceptance is knowing I have a problem. For me it was simply, "I am a sugar addict." Surrender is giving up what I'm addicted to for the rest of my life. If I accept I am a sugar addict, I must surrender it on the altar to God. Obedience is walking out my surrender with the power of God's grace at my back propelling me forward. God won't take the cookie out of my hand, but He will remind me if I ask Him to.

CLOSER TO GOD

The most rewarding part of this journey is getting closer to God. For so many years I was trying, trying, trying to fix my problem myself. When I admitted I had a weakness, I accepted His strength to pull me through.[1]

His strength comes when we totally surrender to Him. Many times mine comes when I am face down on the floor. I get as low as I can to let Him know I am surrendered totally. I invite Him to speak into my life, show me where I'm going astray and show me what I need to do to stop and what I need to start in its place. I have never ascertained God's voice more clearly than after I surrendered sugar, the thing that was more important to me than Him.

Anastacia Maness is a pastor's wife and homeschooling mom who struggled with accepting she was a sugar addict. When she did, though, the change was dramatic.

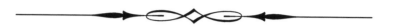

CHANGE STORY
ANASTACIA MANESS

A person not comfortable in their skin hides from cameras. Maybe they hide their fear by taking a few well-posed selfies or hiding behind their children for family portraits. Maybe, just maybe, a family member will manage to get a photo of them when they aren't looking. Sound familiar? That was me.

In November 2012, my family posed for a group picture. My parents were the photographers. I saw the picture and couldn't believe that my clothes fit me so poorly. Needless to say, I wasn't too happy, but I picked the best picture, the one where my kids hid my size, to post online.

Then, my husband and I posed for a picture together. I realized how big I was when I saw the first picture of the two of us. My dad took the second picture. I was pulling on my sweater trying to hide my size. Finally we changed positions and I hid myself behind my husband for the last photo.

Even though I hated those pictures, how I looked didn't make me change my bad eating habits. My husband blamed the camera angle. I blamed my clothes. In those pictures I was 5'10" and wearing a size 18 pants with a stretchy waistband. I really didn't believe I necessarily looked bad as long as I wore the right clothes.

In 2013, I started feeling a change in my health. I couldn't stay awake. I was tired all the time even when I had enough sleep the night before. The only thing that kept me awake was sugar. I ate candy a lot. I kept it in my room hidden from my kids.

I tried to teach my kids moderation. Then, I felt guilty because I didn't have moderation myself. In order to not fall asleep while driving, I kept peppermints with me at all times. I am a homeschooling mom with six children and I had to drive them to many different activities. I knew it wasn't safe traveling half asleep. I wound up having to let my husband do most of the driving. When I did drive I was very tired and ate candy to stay awake.

I'm not addicted to sugar. I can quit any time I want.

Around the end of 2013, I read Teresa's book *Sweet Grace*. After I finished reading I thought that it was a great book. However, I also thought that it didn't apply to me. "I'm not addicted to sugar," I told myself. "I can quit any time I want."

God was trying to show me I had a problem, but I wasn't listening. He was persistent, though. This time the lesson came in a more difficult form. My legs broke out in a rash and my rosacea became unmanageable. I have had rosacea for several years, but it had been manageable. I started doing my own research to find a cure.

Everything I read pointed to processed sugars. Every doctor said to cut back on sugar. Every eating plan said "no processed sugar." I already knew that artificial sweeteners were bad, but I could hardly believe that even "real" sugar was a problem.

My first thought? I can't quit sugar! If God asked me to give up something I really liked would I? This wasn't the first time I had this question come to me. I was taught throughout childhood that anything we put before God is an idol. If I really love God, can I give up my favorite food for Him? I had given up a lot of things before, but never the one comfort food I loved the most — sugar.

Oh, I had cut back on sugar before and had lost a lot of weight, but I didn't give it up completely. When I would stop eating sugar and then start again, the weight I lost would come back, plus some.

There is no Bible verse that says, "Thou shalt not eat sugar." However, I knew it was sugar causing my bad health. I had prayed for a cure to my health problems. I knew His answer was to stop eating processed sugar. I needed to be willing to take the medicine God prescribed. Then, I thought of Teresa's story. She quit eating sugar. I could, too. It wasn't easy.

I QUIT

I quit eating processed sugar at the end of January 2014. I decided if I didn't stop then, I might never stop. I was determined. My husband had a conference the very next week. I planned to take the kids to visit my parents. I called my dad and said, "I'm quitting processed sugar. Please, don't buy me any chocolate milk."

It was my parents' habit to buy chocolate milk for me whenever I visited because they knew I liked it so much. Of course that didn't stop my dad from baking cookies for my kids, but I was proud of myself for resisting the temptation. I have to admit I looked up every recipe on sugar-free cookies I could find while my dad's cookies were baking.

My eyes were only beginning to open to how bad my sugar habit was. My husband used to bring me cookies every day after work. We used to go through a whole package, just the two of us. After I quit eating sugar my husband had to think of something else to bring me. He brought me flowers instead.

Instead of candy for Valentine's Day, he bought me a blender. I know it wasn't that romantic, but I love my blender for mixing smoothies and other recipes. And it did show he loved me because he was supporting my change to a healthier lifestyle

It took me about three weeks to get past the sugar cravings.

Today, any sugary treats given to us are divided amongst our six kids instead of hiding them in our room and chowing down. Now, instead of boxes of chocolates, we eat grapes or almonds for a special treat. I also began replacing bread and pasta with vegetables and salads. Any healthy spread goes on celery instead of bread.

It took me about three weeks to get past the sugar cravings. After just the first week of going off processed sugar, I was more alert. I had no problem driving the four hours to my parents without candy.

I started walking. I used to not be able to walk far at all. I always looked for a bench to sit on whenever we went anywhere. Before I got tired while shopping. Due to the walking, my energy increased. My husband and I started walking two to four miles each day in preparation for a trip to Argentina.

My husband noticed I was more awake while he was driving. I used to fall asleep in the passenger seat every time we went anywhere, even for just a 45-minute drive. Now, I stay awake unless I didn't sleep the night before. With six kids, that happens from time to time.

My taste buds have changed. It's amazing how much better fruits and vegetables taste now. I don't have to have much seasoning at all for food to taste good. I can actually taste the flavors of different herbal teas without any sweetener.

> I am in control of what I eat, instead of my food controlling me.

Of course, the most noticeable change to my friends and family was the weight loss. I started this journey weighing about 219 pounds. I am 5'10" tall. I started off wearing size 18 pants.

By March, I could put on my size 16 pants that I had not been willing to part with. Around June I could wear size 14 pants. I completely skipped buying size 12 and went straight to a size 10. I now weigh 166 pounds. I have lost 53 pounds. I am in control of what I eat, instead of my food controlling me. People still offer me dessert, but I politely turn it down.

When my husband and I went to Argentina, we didn't have our usual foods handy to us. We did well for the first week. We brought healthy snacks on the plane. I refrained from eating desserts, but the more places we visited the harder time I had resisting desserts offered to me. By the second week, I had given up completely on eating healthy. We were doing a lot of walking and I still gained about 10 pounds from that trip.

Every failure is just a learning experience in disguise. The next time we travel to another culture, I will have a plan in place for helping me resist. While there, I realized where I messed up and why. I knew I would have to drop the sugar again as soon as I got back home.

I thought it would be easier the second time since I had done it before. However, the cravings were just as real or maybe even worse. I even had donut dreams. The only thing that helped me through the withdrawals the second time was knowing that the cravings should subside after about two or three weeks of sticking with the process. I fought the mental battle through those two weeks. Today, I am finally free of my sugar addiction and back in control of my eating.

I've learned several lessons from this journey of living without sugar. I have a problem. If I hadn't admitted it, I would have never changed. Denial will thwart change every time. I had to feel the need to change.

NO IN BETWEEN

Once I identified the problem I had to be determined to change. There is no "trying" to get off processed sugar. There is no in between when it comes to sugar addiction. I had to be all in or all out.

Past the sugar withdrawal symptoms, it was easier for me to politely turn down desserts and sweets than it was to go back. That in itself keeps me true to this journey I have chosen with God's help.

I think the hardest part for me is knowing someone else is refraining from eating something just because I am. If I weren't there I know they would enjoy that cookie. I had to know this journey was for me and to not worry about hurting anyone's feelings.

To solve this social problem, I make sure ahead of time that everyone understands they don't have to not eat something just because of me. I also don't have to eat something just because they do. Then, I refuse to feel guilty because I choose to be healthy.

It was hard work to change my eating habits.

For example, my husband prefers the approach of eating sugar in moderation. I can't do that. I know myself too well. I know I will give in too much and be drawn to eat just one more every time. However, I let my husband know that I don't mind him eating it in moderation. I don't feel like I have to just because he does. I should add that my husband has been very supportive and understanding of my decision to eat free from sugar. I believe many more people would stick with their decision to eat healthier and quit eating sugar if they had the support of their families.

I have also learned to prepare ahead. If I am going to a social eating event, I bring something to share I know I can eat. I even fix a little extra in case that's all I can have. There is a vast amount of healthy food available. Once I took that first step and stopped eating processed sugar, including artificial sweeteners, my eyes opened to all the possibilities right in front of me.

There is no denying it was hard work to change my eating habits, but it was possible. God gave me the strength each and every day to do what seemed impossible before. I have made a definite decision to stay away from sugar for good.

What sealed it in my mind that I was indeed a sugar addict was realizing it's not an easy process for me to eat sugar and then try to get back on track. It's more difficult the second time around. It's so much easier, healthier and time efficient to stay away from processed sugar all together.

God knew that about my body. He tried to show me when I read *Sweet Grace*. I was stubborn and prideful though. I thought I had everything under control. He had to use the health issue of rosacea to show me that my body handles sugar differently.

I truly believe God showed me what to do and then helped me take the journey. Even when I went off, He forgave me, dusted me off and set my feet back on the right path.[2] Yes, that's what my God can do.

Before I had head knowledge of the fact that God can help me surrender things you love. Now, I have the experiential and heart knowledge. I know beyond a shadow of a doubt that if God puts it in my heart to give something up I enjoy, He will enable me to do it. I couldn't do it in my strength. I needed His power working through me to strengthen me[3] for the journey.

Anastacia Maness is a preacher's wife, homeschooling mother of six blessings and a writer. When she's not busy counting her blessings she writes about them at http://RockSolidFamily.com where she encourages and strengthens families.

ENDNOTES

1. 2 Corinthians 12:9-10 NIV
2. Isaiah 30:21 NIV
3. Philippians 4:13 NIV

SWEET CHANGE

CHAPTER 12

VICTORY PROCESS

The photo shows a grandmother with six cute grandchildren. The note says, "These are the reasons I want to get healthy." Victory for this woman is something she desires deeply. She has good reasons. Her "why" is firmly in place, but she is afraid she will not be an overcomer.

Grandmothers with weight issues most likely feel some of what she feels. I get emails and messages and comments from people like this every day. They have accepted their issue. They know they need to lose weight and are trying.

Many people, like this grandmother, ask me the inevitable question, "How can I know for sure I will achieve victory in this area?" To answer that we first have to understand what we are asking.

THE BATTLE

The definition of victory is a success or triumph over an enemy in battle or the ultimate and decisive superiority in any battle or contest. It leaves the impression we can be victorious in one battle and lose in another. However, if the battle we are fighting is to become healthy and stay healthy, to gain victory we must change our strategy to begin and continue a long-term lifestyle change.

The truth is we know we have won the war spiritually. However, we're not sure about this battle with unhealthy eating. With His help though, we can also win that war.

Lay the thing we crave on the altar and leave it there.

Acceptance of the issue that caused the problem is the first step. Many people stay stuck here. They have accepted they have a problem and they have tried short-term fixes hoping to go back to business as usual after they gain their version of health, which merely consists of losing a certain amount of weight.

Their own willpower will work to help lose weight for a season, but as soon as the weight has been lost, willpower is put on the back shelf, resolve has been let down and the problems they had before slowly creep back in.

They sigh and say, "See, it didn't work again. I just don't know why God won't give me victory in this area." And they gain the weight back plus more. I know. In my life I've lost 100 pounds at least five times. Every time, except the final time, I gained the weight back plus more.

The real key is the second step, surrender. That's when we lay the thing we crave on the altar and leave it there. We say, "God I'm giving this up for the rest of my life. I want to be healthy to serve and worship you. I want you more than I want that thing."

It's crazy to think we have allowed something as ridiculous as sugar and gluten to take the place of God in our lives. If we crave donuts more than we crave time with God then we have put them in His place.

The only way to combat this is to lay it on the altar and ask for God's help to not pick it up again. We set a firm boundary where processed sugar is concerned. We put something in its place. In my case, it was fruit and exercise. These help keep me grounded and focused on eating to live rather than living to eat.

The third step is obedience to walk out the journey choice by choice, step-by-step holding tight to Jesus's hand, asking His help, inviting the Holy Spirit to remind us when we are going astray and desiring to be held close to the Father's heart.

Nothing tastes as good as freedom feels.

Walking out my victory takes making choices every day. I don't even have to wonder if I will have the chocolate cake for dessert. I will have fruit or, better yet, a protein bar. These choices are ones I know are necessary to keep me free and healthy.

I once was bound in chains of super morbid obesity. Nothing tastes as good as freedom feels. It takes standing against temptation and the tempter's schemes. It takes putting on the full armor of God. It takes being strong.[1] Walking out these steps will bring victory and a chance at many more years to enjoy those grandchildren and great-grandchildren.

Kimberly Weger is well aware of these steps. She struggled for years with health issues only to find the cure was giving up the foods she loved and in that she found victory.

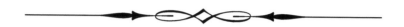

CHANGE STORY
KIMBERLY WEGER

I've never felt very attractive or appealing to the opposite sex. I'm way too short at five feet tall and have always been on the heavy side. Even as a five-pound baby I had Saint Bernard-sized cheeks. I've always had a belly that Santa Claus would envy.

Add to that, in my early 30s I was diagnosed with fibromyalgia. My energy levels were depleted because the Fibromyalgia attacked my legs, especially at night. I would go days with no sleep or I would only sleep two to three hours per night. The pain was debilitating. I had no energy, but I exercised a great deal.

My husband and I own 90 acres and we are "wanna-be farmers." I was busy from 6 a.m. until midnight every day. It was constant run, run, run. The amount of food I ate and my metabolically broken and malnourished body did not allow me to be healthy or at a healthy weight for my small frame.

DIETS AND MY LIFESTYLE

I tried multiple diets. Phen-phen was promising and I have to admit, I looked good in a bikini for the first time in my life. Then, the FDA and a host of doctors reported Phen-phen was very dangerous. So the weight I lost quickly came back with a vengeance and I gained more than I lost.

I tried a nationally recognized weight loss program, but it was a lot of work and I hated counting points. Not to mention, with the appetite I have counting 10 potato chips and calling that a "serving" was excruciatingly painful to manage. I could easily enjoy an entire bag of hot, spicy potato chips with a carton of cottage cheese as a dip.

Many times I waited until my husband went to bed to enjoy a late night snack of chips and cottage cheese, so he would not see my over indulgence.

One of my sisters and I would sweat to the oldies during the day hours while our toddlers played together. Then, in the wee hours of the night we would make a run to the local drive-through for onion rings. We saturated them in mayonnaise, ketchup and salt.

> Eat as much as you want, but don't waste food.

At mealtimes I would continue the charade by cooking what I was taught to be healthy choices for my family. There was always meat, vegetables and potatoes, rice or macaroni of some kind. Then, of course, bread and butter were always on the table.

When I was growing up I was taught to eat what was on my plate. "Don't waste. Eat as much as you want, but don't waste any food." And I ate plenty. I have always felt like I had no shut-off valve where food was concerned. I never had a full feeling and so I could pack it in. Before the kids were tucked in for the night, we would have an evening snack. Sometimes it was nutritious. Sometimes it was ice cream, cake, cookies or popcorn.

Each night I undressed and looked in the mirror. If my husband was asleep, I would tell myself out loud, "You are so fat!" I had no control over my eating habits. I had no control over portion size. Food is an addiction for me. If I had one potato chip, then I would eat the entire bag. One M&M meant the entire 12-ounce bag. The bag of peanut butter eggs in the closet for Easter would call me until I would hide in the closet and eat each individual-sized package. Once I ate two Chicago hot dogs with all the toppings, a brown lunch-bag size serving of fries, a five-pound burrito and a super-sized drink to wash it down.

I always felt if I found one doctor who would tell me what to do and how to do it, I was sure I could do it. I could beat my addictions.

MOTHER'S ILLNESS

Then, in 2008, my mother, Mary Simonson became very sick. She was never one to go to the doctor because she was never sick. She is beautiful. When she was younger many confused her with "Jackie O." However, she and I have at least one thing in common. She too has fought with that belly. She exercised her whole young adult life next to Jack LaLanne on television. She has always walked, biked and now does water aerobics.

She practiced a healthy diet. And she was a fabulous cook. Breads and pastries were her favorite delicacy. She has never liked sweets or soft drinks. She's never given into "snacking." When she got sick and started seeing one doctor after another, it became very frustrating for her when they would tell her, "You are fine." She knew her body. She knew she was not fine.

Somewhere and somehow she was "losing blood." She had blood transfusions and iron infusions. She was hospitalized for being weak and having no energy. Her belly would swell and she would belch non-stop for hours. She would have out-of-this-world backaches. She continued to be iron deficient.

Finally, after months and months of testing, Google searches and digging for answers, her doctor suggested she had celiac disease. At this time we learned that celiac disease is genetic. For her, this diagnosis was a lifesaver, but it also meant a major lifestyle change. It was not an easy change.

This diagnosis was a lifesaver, but it also meant a major lifestyle change.

Our understanding of celiac was limited and the doctor who finally diagnosed her knew only a little more. We began self-learning about the disease. Through our research it was obvious that Mom had an autoimmune deficiency. The nutrients she consumed were not absorbed in her body. Her organs were literally shutting down due to allergens to wheat and other grains. She stopped buying bread.

Many processed foods have wheat and other grains. It wasn't a matter of changing a habit or modifying a diet. It meant no canned goods, no lasagna, no Thanksgiving or Christmas dinner with the big yeast rolls or the beautiful homemade deep dish pies with flaky pie crusts.

Mom tried. She would go like gang busters and eat correctly. It had to be a lifestyle change for her and she took it very seriously. Then, I would come to see her and say something stupid like, "Oh my gosh, you should try this!"

Because of my pressure she would try it. It didn't take long until she was re-hospitalized. My mom was dying and I felt very responsible for her health. It's really hard to go on a radical diet and do it alone. My mom, 250 miles away, was doing it alone.

Quietly and patiently, he told me he believed I had celiac and hypthyroid disease.

So while she was in the hospital, I called her. I promised her I would never pressure her again to try something that was obviously dangerous for her and more than that, I would also "do the diet" with her. No more wheat for me.

Two months later, I met Dr. William Trumbower through my friend Teresa. His nurse made me step on a scale for the first time since my son was born 20 years before.

I cried before the doctor came in the room. I knew I was fat, but I didn't know I weighed 190 pounds. I had been telling a huge fib on my Missouri state license for a long time, but I didn't realize how far reaching that lie was. For my height, that put me in the obese category.

Dr. Trumbower read the result of a series of blood tests I had taken a year before at the request of a female physician whom I had seen for extreme fatigue. When she had read the results to me, she only said that I have a "vitamin D deficiency."

Quietly and patiently he told me he believed I had celiac and hypothyroid disease.

"You are metabolically broken and malnourished," he said.

"My big body can't be malnourished," I joked.

He did not laugh. He knew this was serious. He asked me about my previously reported fibromyalgia condition. I told him about the sleepless nights and my husband sleeping with his legs draped over mine to stop the pain. We discussed my excessive weight gain and inability to lose weight since the birth of my last child and all the diet plans. We discussed my dry hair and dry skin.

He listened like no other doctor ever had. Patting my hand, he said, "You need a lifestyle change, not just a diet."

I told him what I had given up in the way of food in the last two months. He proceeded to give me a list of more foods I was highly allergic to that I should consider eliminating from my diet.

I was actually excited and relieved. Finally, a doctor was telling me what was wrong with me and how to fix it. He also told me how to get rid of the effects of the fibromyalgia. Again it was related to the foods I chose to eat and the foods I chose to eliminate from my diet. Immediately I went to the store to replenish my cabinets and refrigerator. Then, I went home and got rid of the foods that were harmful to me.

> I was actually relieved. Finally, a doctor was telling me what was wrong with me and how to fix it.

Together my mother and I started emailing recipes and links for healthy celiac, which were free from processed sugar, lactose, nightshade vegetables and grains. For me it was a very easy transition. Still, I had to give everything up right now and not do it a little at a time. That also meant that I couldn't "do a little cheat."

My addictions won't allow me to have a little because I still don't know portion control. I still can't say, "Oh, I will have a little and it will be all right." I can't because it won't be all right.

> I still can't say, "Oh, I will have a little and it will be alright." I can't because it won't be all right.

I couldn't believe it when very soon I started sleeping through the night. What an incredible feeling to sleep through the night. I had no pain in my legs for the first time since I was two years old.

Before I knew it I was losing weight. I lost 50 pounds and had to go shopping for new clothes. This time, it was fun shopping. I have energy like never before.

I feel healthy and have remained slim and wonderful for the last four years. I love food. I still overeat, but I overeat on things I know help build my energy. I don't eat what is going to hurt me or debilitate me.

Okay, I admit it, I have cheated twice in almost five years. Both times, I was up all night with a sick stomach and leg pains. It was not worth it.

I still eat free of processed sugar, lactose, grains and night-shade vegetables. Occasionally, I will make myself a hot bowl of rice. It will fill that empty spot.

I know that I don't ever want to go back to an unhealthy lifestyle again. Eating this way has given me health and vitality. It has helped me to sleep peacefully. I am virtually pain free. Why would I ever desire to go back?

Kimberly Weger is a wife, mother of three and grandmother of six. She is a special education teacher and First Steps special instructor. In the summer, she loves her pool, swimming with her five granddaughters and grandson and going on vacation with her mother.

ENDNOTES

1. Ephesians 6:10-11 NIV

SWEET CHANGE

WALKING ON WATER

I used to hate the eight-letter word — exercise. Today, I love my exercise time and guard it carefully. My exercise of choice is water walking. I walk IN the water, not ON it. I exercise five to six days a week for at least an hour sometimes an hour and a half in the water, even in sub-zero degrees. If the indoor pool is open, I go even on the days there are piles of snow on the ground. If not, I exercise to tapes or find a place to walk.

One piece of advice I heard a long time ago was to find some type of exercise I enjoy doing. Problem is, I never liked any type of exercise. I could get A's in all my classes except P.E. How I hated that class. First of all, it was all the way on the other side of creation in a very large high school. Second, I had to change clothes, then shower and dress all over again, plus exercise all in the span of 55 minutes. Worst of all, I had to sweat. I abhor sweat.

The one time I liked P.E. was when we had a semester of swimming. I loved to swim. I could get a good workout, but I never had to sweat. And I can look cute in a bathing suit or at least I could in high school.

On one of the many occasions I went on a diet and lost a lot of weight, the counselor insisted I do some sort of exercise. I was working for University of Missouri at the time and they offered a free water aerobics class at a local gym. I joined and found I really liked it. Like so many other things in my life, I didn't continue with it after the eight-week session was over.

> One piece of advice was to find some type of exercise I enjoy doing. I never liked any type of exercise.

After I had gastric bypass surgery, I was encouraged again to exercise. So I joined our community pool and began attending water aerobic classes. At first, I was concerned about trying to push my massive body into a bathing suit and parading out in front of everyone at the pool.

The pool, though, is a leveling agent. I've always been bigger on bottom than top. Once in the pool, the bottom part is not as readily seen. I enjoyed the water, but I found some of the water aerobic movements taxing on my joints. Plus, I was forever missing the beginning of the class.

As I began to regain weight, I stopped the water exercise all together. It was another on-again, off-again scenario that defined a large part of my life. I was as bi-polar about exercise as I was about the food I ate.

When I started my sugar-free, gluten-free journey about five years ago, I was going to the pool intermittently, whenever I felt like it, which wasn't very often.

My counselor recommended the start-stop method, which said if I stop something, I need to start something in its place. At the beginning, I stopped eating candy.

He challenged me with what I would start. I said, "Exercise." He didn't let me get away with such an elusive answer.

"What kind of exercise will you do?"

"I'll walk in the water." I was proud of that answer, but even I knew it was still pretty noncommittal.

"How is that different from the on-again, off-again water exercise you are currently doing?" I silently kicked myself for revealing that piece of information.

That was a really good question. I didn't want to be nailed down on this one.

"My schedule is really full. I'll just have to do it when I can."

"If you have an appointment, how do you make sure you get to it on time? How do you keep track of your appointments?" He just had to keep pushing, didn't he?

How is that different from the on-again, off-again water exercise you are currently doing?

"I schedule them in my calendar on my phone."

"What would happen if you scheduled exercise like an appointment and kept it every day? What if you saw it like an appointment you are keeping with yourself?"

It was so obvious, it was ridiculous for me to even answer. I just pulled out my phone and scheduled exercise the rest of the week.

At first my plan was to exercise three times a week for 30 minutes, but that first month or so I went every weekday for 45 minutes. I decided I would walk the water track as that did not require me to be there at a specific time.

WALKING IN WATER

The water has a rhythm of its own that soothes my soul. Any cares or worries seem to wash away as I walk. I also find it to be a great time to pray, listen to God's instructions and meditate. It has become a time God knows He has my attention. It's as if He is walking with me. I do at least an hour in the water, six days a week if I am in town and the pool is open.

These days, I'm speeding up and running at least half of the time I'm in the water. The water helps my joints and the pain in what my neurologist calls a broken peroneal nerve in my right leg.

The water doesn't hide the sagging skin on my arms and legs. I'm okay with that, though. I wear the sagging skin gladly. It's a reminder of where I was. It's a place to which I never want to return.

One day as I was running around the water track, a rather upbeat secular song came on the radio. It was as if I could picture Jesus tuck up the bottom of His robe and beginning to dance.

I laughed and said silently, "Jesus do you like that kind of music?"

It was as if He said, "Girl, I invented music."

Jesus and I danced around the track while the lifeguard, who by now knows I'm crazy, just shook his head.

At times it does feel as if I'm walking on water with Jesus right beside me singing and dancing with delight over me.[1]

It has freed me from the tyranny of the eight-letter word — exercise. I now see my time in the water as the beautiful seven-letter word of worship.

I am free. I never desire to go back to bondage again. Never.

Ronda Pickett Waltman feels the same way. Her story is one that involves finding an exercise program which works for her, as well as changing the way she looks at food. Her 109-pound weight loss was definitely life-changing.

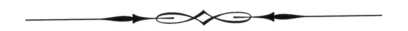

CHANGE STORY
RONDA PICKETT WALTMAN

S ince a very young age I've been overweight. It feels like forever. I just learned to accept it. I have always had a lot of friends and looking back now I am overjoyed because people liked me for me.

We had a very unconventional upbringing in that my mother's parents lived in the same house with my parents and my brother and me. My grandmother's cooking was awesome. She cooked and I ate. It's how she loved us. I tried many different programs to lose weight, but it was my own fault that I didn't stick with them and the weight would come back on. I don't even want to try to count the total number of pounds I lost only to gain them back.

The first program I remember was in junior high or high school and the whole family tried it. It was one of those 1,000 to 1,500 calorie-a-day programs where we measured everything. It just got to be too tiring to do all of that, although I did lose a considerable amount of weight while eating better (not to mention eating less) and doing a lot of walking.

None of the programs worked because I didn't stick with them.

Then, in high school and college I did the Richard Simmons craze. That was fun at first. I also did all the popular videos, "Sweating to the Oldies," etc. The moves were fun and kept my attention and the videos went really fast. Time seemed to fly by. It was one of the few times I actually enjoyed exercise. About 45 pounds was lost doing these and compliments from others really fueled my confidence and pushed me farther.

I moved out of the family home and in with a roommate. We always seemed to have company and parties, and of course with that came food and many carry-ins and potlucks. Not to mention we loved to cook and bake. The weight started coming back on. We were social. Eating is social, so we were eating. I was a happy eater. When in social situations, I ate more.

Basically none of the programs worked because I didn't stick with them. The thing that held me back from change was me — plain and simple. I was actually comfortable in my excess skin and really believed that losing weight would be losing me and who I was. Everyone accepted me for who I was as an overweight person, so why change?

The yo-yo back and forth, gain and lose, got exhausting. I just gave up and thought nothing would ever work. The primary thing that finally propelled me toward change was fitting into clothing. Companies seem to never make clothing in cute styles in the bigger sizes.

The absolute turning point for me, though, was going into a clothing store and finding the cutest sweater. However, I couldn't wear the biggest size they carried, which was a 3X. I just stood in the dressing room and cried. At that moment I decided "I will change." I have power over my life and my weight will not have power over me. My weight will no longer limit me.

I started making a goal to at least lose enough to get into non-plus size clothing. I knew I could not just eat right or just do exercise. I had to do both. Plus, I had to be consistent and not give up.

A good accountability group was important to me. While it's true I needed to want this for myself in order to do it, I also knew I needed to surround myself with positive people who wouldn't judge me. I found that group. They were people to whom I could tell my failures and successes. They would laugh and cry with me. They encouraged me and spurred me on to victory. They became my ongoing change initiators.

EXERCISE AND FOOD

I never liked exercise, but the DVD program called "Walk Away the Pounds" created by Leslie Sansonne remains the best $15 I ever spent. There were three programs — one-mile, two-mile and three-mile. It got rid of the excuses regarding the temperature outside. Those complaints of it's raining, it's too hot, too cold, too dark were no longer relevant.

> Exercise gave me more energy throughout the day because I usually did it first thing.

I did the programs in the comfort of my living room and really enjoyed them. It's mostly walking in place with some kicks, side steps and leg lifts thrown in. Each program gets successively more difficult. I also joined an online group. We encouraged each other.

I never will forget working up to the three-mile program and completing it. I broke down and cried because I did it. Exercise gave me more energy throughout the day because I usually did the program first thing when I got up. It felt good to have done something before going to work. Then, I started doing the programs when I got home at night, as well. The rush of energy I felt was amazing and my sleep was more restful.

I am an extremely social person. I knew my eating habits had to change. Even though I might offend someone for not eating their cooking, I had to do this for me. The way losing weight made me feel was better than any food could taste.

One other habit that seems profound yet never occurred to me before was, if I don't buy it, I don't eat it. Before I had a roommate and we were "feeding" off of each other. Now, I was living alone and responsible for every morsel of food purchased and brought into my home.

I cut out fast food and soda immediately. It didn't seem as difficult as I thought it would be. Sure, there were times of celebration and parties. I put limits on myself and enforced them. I didn't stop eating everything cold turkey, but I managed my portions.

I eat a fairly large breakfast, a moderate lunch and not a whole lot for dinner. I eat dinner by 7 p.m. at the absolute latest and try to avoid late-night snacks. If I do snack, I try to go for lower carb options such as popcorn or nuts

I ate and still eat more proteins and less carbs. I limit my carbs to 45 grams per meal. Foods I alter in consumption amount include rice, pasta, bread and potatoes.

I don't abstain from sugar, but I eat a lot less of it. I try to get it through fruits when possible. I allow myself a little bit of sugar. For me, it's better to have a little of something every once in a while, rather than totally abstaining. If I do abstain, I find a weak moment and eat everything in sight. However, I understand if someone cannot stop with a little, then they should not eat it rather than continuing to stay stuck where they are.

Co-workers were, and still are, extremely encouraging and supportive. They loved me through the entire process. I thank God for these truly amazing people.

AMAZING RESULTS

The journey took four long years and I lost 109 pounds. I went from 254 pounds to 145 pounds, from a size 3X to mediums and larges in shirts. I went from a size 22/24 women's pants to size 8/10 petite. The transformation was a long time coming, but it was totally worth it. I had to come to the realization that I was worth it.

The biggest obstacle to overcome ended up being myself. I would set a goal that was too large to obtain. For me, making smaller goals and reaching them one at a time was best. For example, instead of setting a goal of 100 pounds, I set a goal of 10 pounds, then 10 pounds more. The smaller goals didn't seem so insurmountable. It did get more difficult the less weight I had to lose. The last few pounds seemed to never come off. Yet, I stuck with it. I wanted that goal of reaching 100 pounds and I did it.

> I can walk up a flight of stairs without being out of breath.

Today, life is amazing. I have more energy. I sleep better. I can walk up a flight of stairs without being out of breath. I can walk for miles at a time. It seems funny, but I can bend down and tie my shoes, reach my feet and not be out of breath doing it. Sometimes it's the little things. I never want to take those little things for granted.

I'm thankful and grateful every day for the friends and family who are in my life. One of them is my husband, the love of my life. I met and married a wonderful man who loves me for me. He's encouraging, supportive and pushes me to strive harder every day.

He's become part of my exercise program. We take walks every night after dinner. There are some nights I may not feel like walking. He says, "Let's take a stroll." That ends up being the highlight of my day because we talk during the walk. Sometimes it's silly. Sometimes it's serious, but it's time with him I wouldn't trade for anything.

I admit I used to use time as an excuse. I'd say, "I don't have time for this or that." What I realized is the day is going to go by whether or not I do something, so I might as well do it. I make time to do the things that are important to my health. I've made it a priority to walk at work and use my morning and afternoon breaks to walk with friends. Sometimes we're extremely busy, but we still walk. It always proves beneficial. For health, yes, but we use this time to vent, talk and share.

I know for certain I will never be that person again. I realized I wasn't respecting myself even though I thought I was happy at the time. To be blunt, I was fat and happy. Losing weight was the biggest and most rewarding thing I've ever done. I now feel better than I have ever felt in my life.

Fat and happy was never really true for me. Now, I am lean, energized and joy-filled. I never want to go back to fat and happy.

This is a lifestyle change for me. I will continue to make wise choices about what and how much I eat, exercise and put boundaries in place to keep myself healthy. I never want to go back to the way I was.

Today, I am more in touch with who I am and how God made me. It's interesting how 100 pounds could bury the real me inside my own body. I used to think eating made me happy. I was looking at food all wrong. Food should never be my focus. People and sharing God's love should be my focus.

Fat and happy was really not true for me. I didn't know I could feel any different because I seemed stuck where I was. I learned with vision, a plan and commitment my life can change. Now, I am lean, energized and joy-filled. I never want to go back to fat and happy.

Ronda Pickett Waltman is a senior finance and accounting analyst at the University of Missouri Research Reactor. She enjoys spending time with friends and family, including two very spoiled dogs, as well as reading, walking and cooking. She and her her husband live in Columbia, MO.

ENDNOTES

1. Zephaniah 3:17 NIV

CHAPTER 14

MOVE OVER TEMPTATION

My next-door neighbor has a race car. It looks very cool sitting in his driveway. On Saturday afternoons he fires it up before taking off to the races. I have no idea what type of racing vehicle it is. All I know is that it makes a very loud sound.

Top fuel dragsters produce about 7,000 horsepower. My neighbor doesn't have a top fuel dragster, at least I don't think he does, but still his car has that sound of power. To me it says, "I'm here. Get out of my way. Move or I'll run over you."

It is the opposite of my little four-cylinder Honda that has maybe 117 horsepower. I sometimes feel like it's saying, "I don't know if I'm here or not. I'll move out of your way so you can go around."

Don't get me wrong, I like my little car. It has all the getup and go I need for errands around town, but for the racetrack, a car needs power. Most of the time, though, I don't need to sound louder or wield threats like a 7,000 horsepower engine. I can pretty much take care of things and do fine without that. Or can I? I think I have power over my situation, but do I?

It's interesting that many times the very thing I think I have power over actually has power over me. I don't know how many times I've told myself that I can eat that cinnamon roll because I want it and I need it. After all, we all have to eat, right?

Whether it is food or a myriad of other things, I one day find the very thing I have chosen because I want to have the power to control my emotions and not feel them has power over me. Suddenly, I find myself out of control. I find I have no power. I am weak. I may even find my heart seared to what God says about that very thing. I can't or don't want to hear what He says about what I thought I could control.

> I one day find the very thing I have chosen because I want to have the power ... has power over me.

The deal is, God knew I had this puny horsepower all along, but He didn't leave me at the starting gate. He gave me more than 7,000 horsepower. He gave me all the power in the universe.

"But He said to me, 'My grace is sufficient for you for my power is made perfect in weakness.' Therefore I will boast all the more gladly about my weaknesses so that Christ's power may rest on me. That is why for Christ's sake, I delight in weaknesses, insults, in hardships, in persecutions, in difficulties. For when I am weak, then I am strong."[1]

Wow, God tells me I cannot only sound like a 7,000 horsepower engine, but I can command the road like one, as well. And, I can do it while being in my 117 horsepower body. When I go to Him for help in my time of temptation, He promises to give me a way out,[2] but I have to do something as well. I have to listen to what He says and then do it.

When I first started my healthy lifestyle change, I had one of those extremely stressful weeks. Even though I'd been sticking to my plan and exercising regularly I was ready to give into some kind of eating binge. Just as I was contemplating the same, I heard the still, small voice, the one I had invited to remind me when I was tempted. He said, "You need Me. You do not need food."

I remembered a scripture that spoke about this very thing. I found it. It was the one about God's strength being made perfect in my weakness.[3] It spoke volumes to me. It was what I needed in that moment. It helped me know God's strength will help me overcome. It let me know that God thought of me before time and provided His strength for the times I am weak.

His still, small voice may seem quieter than a four-cylinder engine, but the impact can be greater than that of a high-powered race car when I actually do what He says.

> Once I follow-through with what the Holy Spirit speaks in my heart, it gives me power to withstand the next temptation.

Once I listen and follow-through with what the Holy Spirit speaks in my heart and what I read in the Word, it gives me power to withstand the next temptation. Because I know I was able to be faithful once, with His help I can do it again and again and again.

His power is made perfect in my weakness. I am a top fuel dragster. Move over temptation. I'm coming through.

Only those who have been tempted know what it's like to feel the strength and power of God. One such woman is Donna Falcioni Barr. She was tempted and gave in. What's great about Donna is the fall didn't hurt her. It just made her resolve stronger.

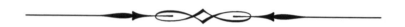

CHANGE STORY
DONNA FALCIONI BARR

Change is sweet when it is happening to us. When it's not, though, it's difficult to watch so many people successfully lose weight. Change would continue to happen to others with or without me. I often wondered why I was unable to reduce in size when others found it relatively easy. After all, the Holy Spirit who gives the fruit of self-control lives inside me. Even people who weren't followers of Christ found weight loss possible.

For 15 years, I had been steadily gaining weight. I chalked it up to a metabolism halt in my mid-40s. I gained 72 pounds during those 15 years. That's about five pounds a year.

If this continued, I would become a diabetic statistic. Each time I had blood work done and my blood sugar checked out fine, I would vow to honor the gift of a second chance to lose weight. All attempts lasted a day or two at best. I just couldn't commit. I didn't want to deny myself the foods I loved. If I denied myself for a day and no measurable results registered, I became discouraged.

Discouragement is a lousy motivator. I would give up until the next alarm sounded. My internal motivation was nil and I knew I needed some external motivation in the form of a mentor. I vowed to do something this past summer to lose the weight.

I was considering a medically supervised plan, but I had the conviction that whatever I did, I wanted to credit God with helping me instead of a program or institution. Another option was what a friend did — she got help through a 12-step group and successfully lost a great deal of weight with the help of a sponsor. Either way, I knew that the personal regular accountability would be key for me.

I had narrowed down the possibilities and counted the financial cost. Then, I read about King Asa. That Bible story made me realize I wanted to find something so that when I successfully lost the weight, I could say, "I did this with the help of the Lord." I didn't want the success to be attributed to a specific program. It needed to be God-centered.

JOURNAL ENTRY

In my journal I had written about how Judah was going to be attacked by Israel. So King Asa[4] decided to send the gold and silver from the Lord's Temple to another neighboring king to make a treaty and prevent the attack.[5] It sounded like a smart plan. However, Asa failed to do one important thing. He didn't rely on God for help. So the seer tells him that the neighboring king was gone.[6] Even though his heart was committed to God, he also failed to ask God to help with a disease he had and only sought out physicians.[7]

I felt a lot like King Asa in that I regularly would seek help from numerous resources. For this weight loss journey, I knew God wanted me to seek Him. My husband assured me that a medically supervised program could be God's means. While I knew this could be true, it just didn't address my desire to attribute success to God instead of a program. Was I looking for yet another way out? Do it perfectly or don't do it at all. I asked God to lead me.

> For this weight loss journey, I knew God wanted me to seek Him.

On June 17, 2014, I received my answer in an email from Teresa. I had been ill with the stomach flu. With little to no appetite for four days, I wondered if a laboratory could isolate the part of the virus responsible for lack of appetite and inject me with it daily. Knowing that wouldn't happen anytime soon, I read on.

The title was 'Risky Sweet Change.'[8] It caught my attention because of the word sweet and the nagging feeling that sugar, too, was also my drug. Well, Sweet Change turned out to be a weight loss coaching and accountability group. It was limited to 50 participants. I worried I might be too late to get in the group? God was clearly in this and it was no surprise I got in.

I had read *Sweet Grace*, Teresa's memoir, and wished I could have her as my personal mentor. This was my opportunity. I could hardly contain my joy. That day, I stopped to thank God for caring for me so much that He honored my desire to include Him in the process along with flesh and blood mentoring.

In my journal entry, I wrote, "I resolved to inquire of the Lord just like King Jehoshaphat. 'Alarmed, Jehoshaphat resolved to inquire of the Lord, and he proclaimed a fast for all Judah. The people of Judah came together to seek help from the Lord; indeed, they came from every town in Judah to seek Him.'⁹ Thank you, Lord, for responding to me so lovingly and specifically."

Since joining the Sweet Change Group, I have lost 35 pounds. I have counted calories using the MyFitnessPal application. My magic number is 1,200 calories a day. I can lose an average of 0.4 pounds a day when I am diligent.

MY HISTORY

When I was a young woman, I was a woman of self-control. I had read a book by Edith Schaeffer in which she challenged women to practice self-control even when it wasn't necessary. So I practiced denial in little things like not eating dessert or not buying something I wanted. When I hit my mid-40s, my metabolism seemed to slow down and my self-denial muscle seemed to atrophy.

My clothes started feeling tighter. I'd ask people in my family, "Do I look like I'm gaining weight?" They would try to assure me I still looked great. Either they were blind or were trying to override my deteriorating self-image. Either way, they did me no favor by being gracious.

Things just continued to spiral downward. Atrophy turned to apathy. I just didn't care any more. The momentary pleasure of taste became more important than the physical consequences.

Anything I tried to fix my weight issue was short-lived. I'm not talking about weeks or months, but hours and days. I had no resolve. Pleasure trumped all. I didn't want to deny myself sweet things. These things failed because I couldn't or wouldn't commit to change. It was too much work. The effects were not instant. Success would breed motivation, but success wasn't happening.

I didn't change because I didn't want to change. I may have said I wanted to lose weight, but I remember confessing to a friend that "apparently" I didn't want to do what it took to make changes in my lifestyle or consumption of food. If I did, I would have already done it.

God's Word showed me my mouth was the source of countless problems in my life. While I went through the motions of gratefulness by thanking Him before meals, I wasn't truly grateful. I felt entitled to eat whatever I desired. I felt deprived if I didn't indulge. I wanted to have a thankful response to each sip and bite and to be more cautious of what my mouth spoke. I had underestimated how difficult this would prove to be, but His Spirit living in me is a constant source of power.

DETOUR

I started the group in July and did well through September losing about 10 pounds a month. Then, as will happen sometimes when you are taking a long trip somewhere, I took a detour. The detour lasted the entire month of October. I started each day by logging my food, but by the middle of the day would opt not to do so. This resulted in a roller coaster ride of gaining and losing the same few pounds.

I feigned busyness and didn't participate in the group often. Others noticed and asked where I was, but they did not push. I know how easy it to take a detour, to never get to your destination. This time, though, would be different. This time, I knew what I wanted. This time, I knew there was a warm,

> I knew they would not condemn me, but support me.

loving, concerned and committed group waiting to welcome me back. I also knew they would not condemn me, but support me.

When I returned to the group, I discovered some things about myself. I decided I would stop entertaining food temptation and whisper or holler, "No!" even if I'm not alone in the room. I've done that at least twice since then and it has helped. I also realized I am becoming free from slavery to desserts. I don't have to have desserts. That freedom is sweeter than the sweets themselves.

I decided to give myself permission to be mildly athletic. I started training to do a 5K in honor of my upcoming 60th birthday. I've never been athletic. I prefer to read, play Scrabble and sip coffee. My preferences are changing because I am changing. I have already signed up and will run that first 5K.

I also noted some non-scale victories related to little dreams I had buried in my heart and mind. I have held on to several clothing items in the hope of fitting into them some day. I have had some of them for 10 years. I tried several on and they fit. So many memories of small failures were redeemed in an instant when I fit into them. Even little successes breed motivation.

I reread my journal entry titled "I Resolved to Inquire of the Lord." I prayed prostrate on the floor before God confessing that I had forgotten the part about His glory. I then reflected on how He has helped me on this journey and thanked Him for His means — His Word; daily personal journal writing; a wonderful app to help me keep track of calories; the Holy Spirit's ministry of conviction of sin, comfort, leading, teaching, help and discernment as well as fruit like self-control; Teresa's mentoring and the support of group members, family and friends.

Losing weight for my own well-being was huge, but doing it in a way that would give me opportunities to honor Him was the real catalyst.

EATING IS AN ACT OF WORSHIP

I wish this process of being set free from ensnaring food was easier for everyone who has the issue with sugar that I do. Teresa reminded me that eating is an act of worship because all that we do is potentially worship — worship of God, worship of ourselves or worship of the devil. I have definitely worshiped myself while eating whatever I wanted for way too long.

I got my resolve back after my detour month. Making God's glory the focus of my choices and my success has been the turning point. I've learned I can worship God with gratefulness and healthy food choices. "So, whether you eat or drink, or whatever you do, do all to the glory of God."[10]

182

Today, brings more opportunities to do the right thing. I am back on the journey. With God's help, I will not regress. I have my resolve back with a conviction that God can redeem anything, even my failures.

Donna Falcioni Barr is a wife, mother of four grown, married daughters and grandmother to five with two more on the way. She teaches English as a Second Language and Preparation for U.S. Naturalization classes. She loves sitting on the floor playing with grandchildren, Scrabble, computers, creating websites, mentoring others, reading, British dramas and studying the Scriptures. She and her husband of 38 years live in Westminster, CA.

ENDNOTES

1. 1 Corinthians 12:9-10 NIV
2. 1 Corinthians 10:13 NIV
3. 2 Corinthians 12:9 NIV
4. 2 Chronicles 15:17 NIV
5. 2 Chronicles 16:2-6 NIV
6. 2 Chronicles 16:7 NIV
7. 2 Chronicles 16:12 NIV
8. http://teresashieldsparker.com/risky-sweet-change/
9. 2 Chronicles 20:3-4 NIV
10. 1 Corinthians 10:31 NIV

SWEET CHANGE

CHAPTER 1 5

SHAME, BARRIER TO GRACE

I was about 11 years old playing hide and seek in the neighborhood. There were four little houses on our end of the street. We ran easily among all the front and back yards enjoying the game. It was a summer night ritual.

Neighbors lounged in lawn chairs in their backyards watching us play. Sister Forsee sat on her screened-in front porch brushing the long white hair that she kept up in a bun during the day. I'd go in and volunteer to dust her statues. She had many angels and other ceramic items. They had been collected over a lifetime. They each had a story, which she loved to share.

Mikey's parents lived in the last house. We lived in the first house. There was a lot of visiting back and forth. My mother and Mikey's mother loved to talk and play cards. It was a neighborhood where we weren't afraid to be out at night.

As one of the oldest kids, I was always first back to base and rarely had to be "it." This evening, though, I was it. It was late afternoon. The sun was going down to cool the heat of the day. All was right with the world.

I was having a great time, not really worried about whether I could find everyone or not. Not worried about winning the game, just enjoying the atmosphere of calm, serenity and familiarity. I counted to 100 and then yelled, "Ready or not,

Out of the corner of my eye I saw Mikey, the youngest boy, run around the corner. He saw me see him. He knew he wouldn't be able to get away. He knew he would be caught. Perhaps that's why he yelled it. Perhaps it was just to be mean. Perhaps it was to throw me off course so he could get to the base.

"Crisco, Crisco, fat in the can. You couldn't catch me no matter how fast you ran," he yelled. And he laughed a mocking laugh.

If he was trying to make me mad, it worked. If he was trying to get me to leave the game, that worked too. If he was trying to make me ashamed … Bingo, that really worked.

> Crisco, Crisco, fat in the can. You couldn't catch me no matter how fast you ran.

I stomped inside angry at the tauntings of a three-year-old. I vowed never to play with the little kids again. Of course, they didn't care. They went on playing. As a matter of fact, his plan of getting me to leave base so he could come in worked too.

I told myself I wasn't fat. In reality I wasn't a chubby kid, but I sure felt fat. "Crisco, Crisco fat in the can" churned around and around in my head for decades after that incident.

I know now that it wasn't Mikey's words so much as the accuser's words who used that situation as a launching pad to build a wall of shame in my life. I was guilty of eating more than I should have, even as a kid. I'd sneak candy and cookies whenever I could. It was a comfort to me.

In reality, there were things in my life that weren't always as idyllic as that summer night prior to Mikey's taunts. My mother had some emotional issues that left me in charge of the house and my brother and sister a lot of the time. I learned early that food would comfort me and make the pain go away for a little while. And so I ate whenever I could, preferring candy, cookies, cakes, sweet breads and donuts over anything else.

> Jesus is grace personified, asking for me to turn from the things causing me guilt and shame.

The guilt of what I did, turned into shame. The shame said, "You are what you did. You are fat. You are shameful. You are a horrible donut monster." Shame followed me. I never could quite shake it. I never really understood until much later, even after becoming a Christian, that grace is the trump card that does away with shame.

Jesus stands as my Advocate who says, "Maybe you have done some things wrong. Let's look at those and talk about what we can do to work on them."

For some reason the screaming voice of shame, the accuser, was much louder than the calm, quiet voice of the Advocate who gave me advice and answers. Jesus is grace personified, asking for me to turn from the things causing me guilt and shame.

Here's the thing about grace. I understood when I accepted Christ as my Savior at age seven, I got grace for all my sins, past, present and future. I just figured if I followed all the rules the church laid down, I'd not have future failures.

I didn't consider eating whatever I wanted as a sin. The church didn't talk about overeating as sin. Sure, there were sermons about drinking and premarital sex as sin. However, those overly large preachers never talked about gluttony. Eating as much as one wanted was the acceptable thing to do in the Christian circles I grew up in.

I knew, even as a child, I had an unnatural love for things made with processed sugar. I was like a person gone mad when I had candy. I looked forward to times like Christmas, Easter and Halloween when I could have unlimited candy. I would eat every bite I could for fear others would eat it before I did.

OVEREATING

It reminds me of a foster son we had who would go to the refrigerator and stuff down an entire package of bologna in a single gulp and still go back for more. I understood his unlimited need for food. In essence, I had the same need only for things made with sugar. I felt bad limiting his intake of any food when mine was so out-of-control.

It was interesting to me that God seemed to continue to bring individuals with food issues to our home. Didn't He understand I couldn't help them? Of course He did. I believe He was bringing them to me to be a mirror to my own life.

In essence, it did work. I had one definite moment of change on this journey. However, there were many minor moments throughout my life. It takes a lot of steps to make a journey. These were just some of the steps along mine that pointed me to what I needed to do. I needed to do exactly what I was doing with foster children who couldn't stop eating.

In one instance, we got a physician's order to put locks on our refrigerator and pantry. The problem was I had the key. Oh yeah, this was for the foster son, right? But what was God trying to tell me? When we had three foster daughters with weight issues, I stopped buying chips, cookies and sodas, at least for the kitchen pantry and refrigerator. However, there was a small refrigerator in my room and drawers and closets where I could hide my stash.

HOW IS THIS A MIRROR?

What was God trying to tell me? What was the mirror I was looking into? Who was the face staring back at me? What limits was I willing to place on myself? And if I couldn't place those limits on myself what right did I have placing them on others?

By this time I had gained up to 430 pounds. I never really saw weight gain as sin. God, however, does see anything we put before Him as sin. I had definitely put comfort foods, before Him. Putting it that way means for me, it was sin. It especially was because I chose to disregard what God showed me in 1977. When I had prayed God showed me my issue was with processed sugar and if I would stop eating it and start eating more fruits, vegetables and meats I would lose weight.

I'm not sure why I couldn't understand that exactly what God said, is what He meant. "Stop eating sugar." He didn't mean stop for a season, which is what I tried to do many times with various diets. He chose His words wisely. He meant stop. If I would have stopped, the cravings would have stopped and I would have been able to control my weight.

It took over 30 years and coming to the end of my rope before I followed what He said. I was in disobedience all of that time because I didn't follow what I know He told me to do.

> For years all I could see was a wall of shame built of processed sugar and flour.

Through this journey I've learned quite a few things about grace. Here are a few. God's grace covers me no matter what I do wrong.[1] God's grace sent Christ to the cross so I don't have to live in guilt and shame.[2] God's grace propels me forward when I repent of things I have done wrong.[3] God's grace tells me I am worthy of God's love because I am in Christ and He is worthy.[4] God's grace is present so I can receive the gifts He has designed for me to be able to complete His assignment on my life.[5]

For years all I could see was a wall of shame built of donuts, cakes, cinnamon rolls, processed sugar and flour. I couldn't see God's grace. There was this giant barrier I had built between God and me. It felt like He was jumping up and down, standing on His tippy toes trying to peek over the mountain of junk food, waving His arms and saying, "Hey, I'm over here. Just tell this wall to move and it will. Then, you can see Me completely."

Moving the wall, even if I could figure out how, was really, really scary because it had become my comfort zone. I don't know what wall others have built between themselves and God. I know I definitely had a wall that God in His grace removed from my life.

God is grace. He longs for a solid connection with us. He doesn't want the wall of shame to define us. He would rather He define us. Shame shuts us down and makes us ineffective in the Kingdom. He wants us to ask forgiveness for our wrongs, repent and move on to do the work He has called us to.

He knows us. He knows our human tendencies. We will fail because we are not perfect. To do the work, He has given us a myriad of gifts so that we might serve others.[6] It's a plan only God could design. He had our backs before we even messed up. What a God we serve.

> God is grace. He longs for a solid connection with us.

This next story is about a woman I just met this year. The weight of shame she felt over something she had done in her life built a huge fortress between her and God's grace. She, like me, could only see her shame. Year after year, she piled layer after layer of shame on herself. Mostly she kept her weight under control with an eating disorder.

After a bottom-of-the-barrel experience, Nora Ann Treguboff Saggese finally reached up to grab hold of the strong arm of God's grace. It has taken hard work and perseverance, but one by one the layers are being removed and the walls of shame are tumbling down to reveal the majesty of His grace.

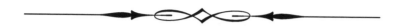

CHANGE STORY
NORA ANN TREGUBOFF SAGGESE

These verses describe my life journey. "Are you tired? Worn out? Burned out on religion? Come to me. Get away with me and you'll recover your life. I'll show you how to take a real rest. Walk with me and work with me — watch how I do it. Learn the unforced rhythms of grace. I won't lay anything heavy or ill fitting on you. Keep company with me and you'll learn to live freely and light."[7]

There was never a time in my life I didn't know God, but it was a long journey towards an intimate relationship with the One who loves me more than I will ever know. The Lord relentlessly and passionately pursued me. As He pursued me, I would slowly surrender and release the pain.

> Shame used to be my middle name. I was on a mission to prove to God I was worthy of His love.

Shame used to be my middle name. I was on a mission to prove to God I was worthy of His love. Because of numerous circumstances in my life, I struggled with overeating, binging and purging, otherwise known as bulimia.

It is a terrible eating disorder I battled for more than 37 years. Today, I am walking toward freedom as I get closer and closer to my God and King. I am learning I am His. I am royalty.

It has not been an easy journey and continues still.

My mother had a breakdown during the first trimester of being pregnant with me. She was taken to a mental hospital where she was put on strong drugs and had shock therapy treatments. At one point while she was carrying me she fell down 14 stairs and broke her leg.

My father tells me that the doctors wanted to terminate the pregnancy through a therapeutic hysterectomy because they feared I would be retarded and mentally handicapped. They did not know how a baby could survive unscathed in utero after a mother had gone through so much. My dad said he would trust God and receive whatever gift he was given. My mother says I was a miracle baby as I was born without a problem and am gifted in many ways.

> I wasn't hidden from God when I was made in this secret place.

There is much talk today about how babies can hear before they are born — respond to music, arguments, the sound of a mother's voice reading to them. All my life I felt I had to prove that I deserved to live. I wonder if it stemmed in some way from this talk of aborting me.

God, though, created every part of me. He knit me together in my mother's womb. I know I am fearfully and wonderfully made. Everything He does is wonderful and so am I. I wasn't hidden from God when I was made in this secret place. I was woven together in the depths of the earth. He saw my unformed body. Every day of my life was ordained by Him.

Every day was written in His book before a one of them came to pass.[8]

I know that today, but as a child I felt like a castoff. My mother and father divorced and I was left with my mother and her parents. Divorce and my mother's illness were two strikes against me.

I grew up in a closed ethnic religious community with emphasis on rules, right and wrong and a confusing theology. One did not question authority. Only those of our Russian heritage were allowed in our church, so I could not invite friends to the service. When I asked about this I was told there were enough of "our own kind" who are lost without bringing any more in.

> In school, I was bullied for being fat. I was just a normal, chubby girl who developed early.

I was an outcast because my mother was divorced and our family was broken. So I was allowed to go with my friends to their churches. This is where I accepted Jesus at age 7.

Around this time, my mother went to Los Angeles, two hours away, to get a job and start a life for us. She promised to return for me. I stayed with my grandparents. While she was in LA, she had a full-blown breakdown and I didn't see her for six months. I was sad and felt abandoned. This is when I learned to medicate with food.

In school, I was bullied about being fat. In reality, I was just a normal, chubby girl who developed early. My best friend was a boy. I remember hearing someone say that I would be barefoot and pregnant by the time I was 15.

In my adolescent way of thinking I decided I needed to come up with a disease to not draw attention to myself. I made up symptoms for diabetes. I played it so well, the doctor decided to put me on a high sugar diet for a week to see if I had diabetes. In one week, I gained 15 pounds.

I didn't have diabetes, but that set me up for sugar addiction. I ballooned up to 245 pounds fairly quickly. This crazy way of eating continued through high school.

Because of my weight, I had friends who were boys, but not boyfriends. I didn't date. I didn't go to the prom. I didn't do any of the things normal teenagers did. I ate, studied and worked.

When I was 18 and graduating from high school a doctor told me, "You are on a treadmill to die." He put me on a balanced meal plan and I dropped down to 185. It was just enough to be healthy, but still gave me insulation to protect myself from sexual advances. My desire was to be successful in college and make something of myself.

There was always a fear of boys taking advantage of me and always cautions by my grandfather of that happening. Getting pregnant out of wedlock was not tolerated. One would get married or be cast out of the community.

BIG MISTAKE

I didn't want to get pregnant, but I did want a relationship. No one wanted to date the fat girl, but when I was 20 a friend set me up with a guy from our Russian community. Later I would learn he only went out with me because I was a virgin and thus, an easy target.

I was a good girl. I never did anything to disappoint my family. I was a naïve farm girl. As soon as I started dating him, I knew what he wanted. One night he date-raped me. When that box was opened, it had serious implications.

> Because of the fear of shame, I made a decision that went against all my values and beliefs.

I stayed with him, because I believed my virginity should be a gift to my husband. So in my mind I had to marry him. I continued to date him. He continued the subtle brainwashing process. I allowed myself to be mentally and sexually abused by him.

It seemed my lot in life to marry him even though I knew I didn't love or trust him. And he for sure didn't love me. He would even say, "I lust you," but never, "I love you." I felt I didn't deserve anyone else. I would have to settle.

Then, the day I feared came. I was pregnant. He didn't want to marry me. I was staunchly against abortion and had written a college paper on it. One illustration I used in the paper, which he had proofread, said, "Children are not teeth that you just have pulled out."

When I told him I was pregnant, he said, "I guess you'll have to pull out one of your teeth."

Scared and alone I had an abortion. He didn't support me and I couldn't tell anyone in my family. Because of the fear of shame, rejection, disappointment and letting my family down,

I made a decision that went against all my values and beliefs. I aborted my child.

What I did tormented and haunted me for years. Everywhere I went, the pain of what I did followed me. I began punishing myself. It began with eating to anesthetize the pain. Concerned with additional weight gain, I had read somewhere about what seemed like a magic fix. If you eat too much, just throw it up. This opened the door to a serious struggle with bulimia.

The only thing in my life I felt like I could control was what I put in my mouth. And after I put it in my mouth, the only way I could control not gaining weight was to throw it up. The bulimia advanced to being very severe. I was going to college and living in an apartment.

My bulimia was completely out-of-control. I might go and get orders of eight burgers and fries, three dozen donuts, packages of cookies and a gallon of ice cream. Or I'd get pancake mix and make 25 to 40 pancakes. I would eat until I threw up. There is a high that is connected to binging and purging. It is also very addictive.

Because we didn't have the greatest plumbing system, I got five-gallon paint buckets and seven to 10 times a day I would fill those with purging. Then, I'd get a large strainer and strain and flush. I'm being graphic to make a point. It was a mess. I was on scholarship. I was an intern, nanny and full-time student with this secret life.

This opened the door to a serious struggle with bulimia.

I would look normal to anyone I met or who knew me. I was in control in front of people. I maintained my weight at 180. I had a fear of dying of obesity, but eating helped me stuff the pain. Then, the purging seemed to release the pain.

It was doing horrible things to my body. And in reality it wasn't helping the emotional pain of what I'd done by aborting my baby.

I went overseas on a scholarship to Moscow and then Rome. One time in my dorm room, I remember purging. It resulted in bleeding from my throat. It scared me. I prayed and asked God to help me and I stopped my struggle with bulimia for a several years.

I met my future husband in Rome. He was the first man ever to like me for me. He was he first man to tell me he loved me. Before we got married, I maintained my weight by doing a very controlled form of dieting, which again would not last for the long haul.

I did stop the full-fledged bulimic activity, but I would have relapses when I got angry, frustrated or overwhelmed. A relapse was often a one-time incident, never full blown like in college. For many years I maintained the weight within 20 pounds. I'd gain and lose, gain and lose and repeat again.

MAJOR RELAPSE

I realize for most of my life I had still been controlling my eating by my own power with either controlled dieting or occasional relapses. So it shouldn't have been any major surprise to me that five years ago, when it seemed I couldn't control everyone and everything around me, I went into a major bulimic relapse.

The bottom seemed to fall out of my life in every area. My two sons were at that point where they were making their own way. I had plans for them and wanted them to fit in the box I had made. However, I learned I cannot control or stuff others into my molds. Still, I so wanted to.

> I felt like a failure, a terrible wife, a terrible daughter, a terrible mom, a terrible teacher.

Then, my mother had some health difficulties and I needed to help her. She lived down the street in a separate apartment, but I began having to take care of her and check on her every day. There were times when she yelled at me and called me horrible names. It was overwhelming trying to mother my mother, something I have done for most of my life.

My husband had been diagnosed with a brain tumor 13 years before this. I began realizing how our dreams seemed to be dying. After 30 years of teaching, everything began changing in my profession. I felt out of date and obsolete in a profession I loved.

The bottom line was that I felt like a failure — a terrible wife, a terrible daughter, a terrible mom, a terrible teacher. I stepped down from all ministries because I did not want to damage others. Everything crashed down on me. Everywhere I looked there were constant pressures. I began to anesthetize with food again. Once again I began trying to control what I ate with purging.

I began seeing a counselor, but was still involved with occasional bouts of bulimia. At one point I passed out from the purging and hit my head on the toilet. Another time I drank hydrogen peroxide, passed out and was unconscious.

I had to have reconstructive surgery on my jaw and teeth because of the damage from hyrdrochloric acid, which is made in the stomach. When I would regurgitate, this acid would come up from the stomach and erode enamel on my teeth. Over time the cumulative effects caused many health problems.

On the outset, bulimia looked like an easy solution for eating whatever I wanted whenever I wanted it, but there were at least five times I could have died from what I was doing to my body.

Two years ago, I had a sore festering on my leg for several months, which I ignored. It was sepsis and by the time I got to Urgent Care they said I was two hours away from the poison getting to my heart. It took a month or more for me to heal and get my energy back from that. I was well aware of how close a call I'd had.

BECOMING ROYALTY

April 7, 2014, is a day I will never forget. My husband put out a large aquarium out for me to take to my classroom the next day. He set it in the driveway next to my car. At 5:30 a.m., when I left out the door for school, it was dark.

I didn't see the aquarium. I tripped and fell into it. Glass shattered everywhere. I was on my knees in a pool of blood. I could feel the pieces of glass. How many people can trip over an empty aquarium and land on their knees? That was the moment my life changed.

I had built a mighty fortress to protect myself. My Father knew my pain. He heard my every cry. The pain and the walls seemed to come tumbling down.

> I wanted the obsessive throughts of food to stop.

My first thought was, "Oh no, this cannot be happening. Who will teach my class?" I was bleeding and in pain, yet I couldn't think of myself or the damage. Nineteen stitches later, I was home for three weeks with time to think, read and listen to the Father's still, small voice.

I prayed for an answer. I was weary of being sick and tired. I wanted to reclaim my life. I wanted the obsessive thoughts of food to stop. My deep desire was for balance, order and clarity. This was my moment. I hit bottom.

My Father had me on my back during Holy Week. As I examined my life, I knew something had to change. I knew the reasons for past failures and I needed a plan.

The plan had to include deep emotional healing, exercise and a food plan. God helped me to say, "Hello. My name is Nora and I am a food addict. I am powerless. I need a Savior."

Sugar and gluten were my drugs of choice. Instead I decided I needed three meals a day with two high-protein snacks. I knew I had to get away from my addiction to food before I could get to the truth of my pain. A series of events and an elephant picture with Teresa's blog post led me to the Sweet Change Weight Loss Coaching and Accountability Group.

I am immensely grateful for July 1, 2014, the starting date of my Sweet Change journey. Weight loss measured in pounds has been a slow, steady process. I have lost 24 pounds and am not far from my goal. I walk with friends and work out with a wonderful coach. Physical exercise is a gift on this journey.

My deep desire was for balance, order and clarity.

The loss of emotional pain has been immense. Each day I recover a part of my life and with each moment I learn the unforced rhythms of grace. Keeping company with my Jesus has been a gift that keeps on giving. The best is yet to come.

I am filled with gratitude as I experience daily transformation by the renewing of my mind through God's Word, His love letter to me. Reading the Word of God and sitting in silence help me to hear the sweet voice of my Savior. I am also learning to forgive, which is setting me free from captivity. This also keeps me away from food.

If someone would have told me that cravings would cease, voices would be turned off and my mean and angry outbursts would end, I would have thought it a fairy tale, given my history. However, all of this and more has happened as I surrendered processed sugar and gluten to God.

Free at last. Free at last. Thank God Almighty, I am free at last! How do I know that it's real this time? The noise has stopped. For the first time in 50 years. I can look at my reflection and like what I see. I matter. I am valuable, dearly loved and the King of Kings' princess.

I hadn't believed this since the age of seven, when the little broken girl turned to food out of need for comfort from her pain. I will never go back to Egypt — to bondage. Each day brings new treasures. Each day is an amazing gift. My desire is to be the fragrance of Christ to the hurting. I desire that strangers watching me might be transformed by my example. I have a dream — to write my full story and to coach women who are emotionally and physically wounded.

As I write this, I weep. Nearly 50 years ago a little girl turned to food for comfort. For many years, I would struggle for sobriety. Today, I am free. I have the tools to remain free. My past failures do not define me. I listen to His still, small voice. My accountability group walks with me and where He leads, I will follow.

What is the difference this time? I have Teresa, a coach who listens, and a wonderful tool she calls stop-start. I have a group of faithful friends and an amazing life coach and a trainer who challenges me to new fitness levels.

I am royalty because I belong to God who humbles me and lifts me into His presence at the same time.

I live joyfully because I know who holds the future. I am excited. I love my life. It's full of real stuff like a husband, kids, work and a mother whom I care for, but at the center there's my Father God. His love for me is unfathomable.

Today, one song keeps playing in my head. It's called, "Royalty" by Kimberly Rivera. It talks about shattered dreams and the realization we matter to God. I love just knowing I am royalty because I belong to God who humbles me and lifts me into His presence at the same time.

I never felt I was worth anything, but God speaks to my heart and tells me I matter. I have worth. I have value. I have purpose. I am royalty.

Nora Ann Treguboff Saggese is a wife and mother of two adult sons. She has been a teacher for 34 years. She enjoys outdoor exercise especially hiking and running. She loves intercessory prayer, inner healing ministry, art to heal, praying in color and digesting the word of God instead of sugar. She lives in Downey, CA.

ENDNOTES

1. Ephesians 1:7-8 NIV
2. John 3:16-18 NIV
3. Romans 5:20 NIV
4. Romans 3:23-26 NIV
5. 1 Peter 4:10 NLT
6. ibid.
7. Matthew 11:28-30 MSG
8. Psalm 139:13-16 NLT

CHAPTER 16

EXTRAORDINARY FUTURE

We have extraordinary futures. Some days, I dare to dream that is true, but there are days I don't. Several years ago, I was more than a little down on myself. I was hungry, angry, lonely and tired. There was no dreaming of great things, only slogging through the daily grind of life and not enjoying it.

I was hungry because I was trying to stop consuming mainly protein shakes and starting to eat real food, but I didn't have a real plan for that besides stopping the thing that was keeping me from being hungry.

I was really mad at myself. Okay, I was having a pity party. I was frustrated for allowing interruptions to guide my day rather than my intended values. Both the pity party and the frustrations were a not very well veiled form of anger.

When I get busy, I tend to become introspective which leads to a type of loneliness. I wasn't taking time for deep, meaningful discussions because I was, well, busy. I was getting into exercise, but that was just making me more tired. I hadn't gotten to bed as soon as I would have liked most nights. Again, I blamed busyness and looming deadlines.

I had all of the ingredients ripe for backsliding into an abyss. I was Hungry, Angry, Lonely, Tired. The acronym HALT is appropriate because for an addict, these are ingredients for relapse.

One way I define an addiction is a place I have gone that has given me an easy sense of comfort, but has been impairing my life. For me that is eating sugar and flour. I was in the beginning stage of giving these up. However, I wanted a quick fix, a way to anesthetize the discomfort I was feeling.

> I had all the ingredients for backsliding into an abyss.

My brain recognized this was not a good place to be. I needed a different kind of relief; something positive that would be long lasting and not life limiting. I began to think about someone in scripture who was in a similar situation. It took me awhile to search, but I found what I was looking for.

"Why are you cast down, O my inner self? And why should you moan over me and be disquieted within me? Hope in God and wait expectantly for Him, for I shall yet praise Him, Who is the help of my countenance, and my God."[1]

At that point I certainly needed help with my countenance. No doubt about it.

Compared to all of my puny problems, David, the writer of the Psalms, had much larger ones. He ran from King Saul, committed adultery and murder, faced national problems, fought countless battles, was surrounded by enemies, lost a child as a baby and lost more children as adults. Yet, despite all of David's problems and faults, he was called a man after God's own heart.

In the book *Mother Teresa's Secret Fire,* Joseph Langford writes: "Wherever we are, with whatever talents and relationships God has entrusted us, we are each called not to do what Mother Teresa did, but to do as she did — to love as she loved in the Calcuttas of our own life." What he was saying was that not all of us are called to the physical city of Calcutta, but we all have situations in our own lives that may seem as difficult as those in Calcutta experience.

I thought about my own "Calcutta" of recent weeks. My "hungry" wasn't because I had nothing to eat. My "angry" wasn't because I had no place to live. My "lonely" wasn't because all of my family and friends had died of malnutrition. My "tired" wasn't from begging in the streets of Calcutta.

Yet, all of those Mother Teresa helped were in those situations. It's amazing that she was able to go on day after day helping the most desperate of humanity. She knew only the light of Jesus touching them could bring any hope into their darkness.

By comparison my "Calcutta" was ridiculous.

King David's "Calcutta" was different, but there were times he was hungry, angry, lonely and tired. Just read the Psalms. His desperation is there, but also his confessions and his praises of an almighty God.

By comparison my "Calcutta" was ridiculous, really. Just thinking about it was, laughable. It helped me re-frame my situation. It helped me accept where I was. It helped me own my life. It helped me want to reach for more, to be more, to embrace more fully who I am and who I am destined to be.

It's a little like Reepicheep says in *Voyage of the Dawn Treader*: "Extraordinary things happen to extraordinary people. Perhaps you were made for an extraordinary future." Perhaps, indeed.

Each person was created for an extraordinary future. I know this because God tells us He has plans for us that are good and not disastrous. They are plans for a future and a hope.[2]

One such woman is Heather Tucker. She has gone through some great difficulties in her life. God, however, is moving her, as He does each of us, to an extraordinary future.

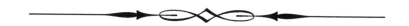

CHANGE STORY

HEATHER TUCKER

My weight gain was triggered by an abusive husband, but the root of it was embedded in me years before. My mindset towards most major life events has contributed to my inability to lose weight.

During my teen years, I was a normal weight. Once I went through puberty, I developed in such a way that I caught the attention of many onlookers, both envious women and lustful men. It didn't take much attention for me to realize my value was in my body, a lie that I fight against every day of my life, even now.

When I started college in 1993, I started working out at the gym daily to fine-tune my voluptuous body, which was becoming quite sculpted. I was at a point in my life where without realizing it my self-worth and heart were damaged. I continued the same destructive lifestyle, while trying to change my spirit.

MARRIAGE

It was then the Holy Spirit beckoned me to Him. I became a Christian, but I got into a relationship that nearly ruined me. I married an abuser. From this hell-driven relationship, God has blessed me with an incredible daughter who is now 15 and loves the Lord with all her heart.

After I delivered my daughter in 1999, I immediately began working to lose the baby weight by eating healthy and exercising daily. This was successful for a while, until my husband transitioned from emotional and mental abuse to physical abuse.

Eventually, I left him when my daughter was six months old. I thought I would continue to lose the baby weight, cut him out of my life and move on. Little did I know the terror would not be over. Instead, he continued attacking me with vile threats and he stalked me. Still, I had to allow him to take my baby for visits. We had to exchange her at the police department because of his threats to me. I was scared. I had a lot of fear, which set up my desire to self-protect.

The weight came back on plus more. I had gained 60 pounds during my pregnancy. I continued gaining and put on another 30. My goal now is to lose a total of 80 pounds and most importantly, become healthy both physically and emotionally.

It's strange to know I was trying to self-protect with food. I thought if I could hide my body under the weight, then men wouldn't be lusting after me and bad things wouldn't happen to me anymore. Little did I know, my food choices would catch up to me.

Over the years I would get tired of feeling unhealthy, lethargic and tired and begin to cut out junk food and carbs. I would lose 15-20 pounds, begin to feel better and then go back to eating.

I always knew what I was doing wasn't giving me the desired results.

I lived consumed by fear, which was the lie of the enemy to keep me in bondage. It was not about the weight, it was about receiving healing for the hurt and pain. My past hurt and pain was the root and the weight gain and lack of weight loss was the fruit of that root. Only God could extract that root if I let Him. Only He could be my Champion, my Knight in shining armor, my Comforter, Defender, Provider and, most of all, my Protector.

I always knew what I was doing wasn't giving me the desired results. I knew what it took to get the results. Trust God with my broken heart, allow Him to heal me, trust myself to make godly decisions that I believe with my whole heart and give Him control by giving up the fear that so entangled me[3] into keeping the weight.

The combination of counseling and the Holy Spirit ministering to me helped me to trust that He wants good things for my life. He has a plan and a purpose for my life that does not include bondage from past pain, hurt and abuse.

My life verse says it best. "'For I know the plans I have for you,' declares the Lord, 'plans to prosper you and not to harm you, plans to give you a hope and a future.'"[4] The verses that follow declare that the Lord promises when I call upon Him in prayer, He will listen to me and answer me. I will find Him when I seek Him with all my heart.[5]

I recognized that I am nothing without God. All my attempts to lose weight and read faith-based self-help books failed because I still had to call on Him. I had to humble myself before the Almighty King who heals me, then change could start.

EVERYONE ELSE FIRST

I live in a multigenerational household raising my daughter and taking care of my mom when her health problems impair her physically, putting their needs before mine. I was raised that way — that strong women take care of the family. I was taught it's not about my needs, but the family's.

Due to many events that have culminated over the last few years, I decided to take off time from work this summer and focus on me. I got to spend lots of time with my daughter, finish my degree and begin therapy, where I worked through different issues I was dealing with. There was only one thing left — the root of my weight problem. It was time to pick off the fruit, one by one and allow the Holy Spirit to prune me physically and emotionally to become the godly woman He called me to be.

I cried out to God and said, "God, I need help! I know how to eat right, I know how to exercise and which exercises my body responds to. I know all this, but I need help. I need someone who understands. I need someone to guide me on this journey. I can't do it alone. I can't do it with just you Lord. I need support!"

Within about two weeks, the Lord brought Teresa to me. We go way back. She was my spiritual mama when my mother was battling cancer and she's never left me, even though we moved back to southwest Missouri. I have been on Teresa's email list since it began. I stumbled across her weight loss coaching and accountability group, Sweet Change, which was starting.

I said I would pray about it, knowing this was an answer to prayer. I did that because I was afraid. I laid down my fear at the feet of Jesus and jumped in. While working the program and studying the Word, I read her book, *Sweet Grace*. It was like she was in my head from birth. I received so much healing from her transparency and brutal honesty. I was ready to conquer this evil bondage called fear. My weight loss would follow.

STRENGTH AND HEALTH

My entire life changed as I turned the corner. I had to learn to put me first, not in a selfish manner, but in a healthy way that strengthened me to be strong for my family on a daily basis. That included my physical health, in addition to my emotional and mental health. I knew it was God's will for me to be healthy, to stop abusing my body with food.

I am just in the beginning of this journey. I have ambitious goals to lose the weight and I want to never go back once I have. In the past when I made an unhealthy decision, I would just stop working on losing weight and eat whatever I wanted. This time, I've learned to forgive myself, ask for the Lord's strength and try again.

The root of my weight gain and lack of weight loss is fear. It is fear of what others will do to me because of how I look and fear of me again believing my value is in my body. The Lord is delivering me from these fears.

> The root of my weight gain and lack of loss is fear.

Every layer or pound that I shed is another issue from which God is healing me. Every pound that comes off gives my Healer an opportunity to work a deeper level of healing in me. Once this root is completely extracted, the fruit will be removed and the ability for it to return will not exist. I must crucify my flesh daily.[6] As I decrease, He will increase.[7]

My life has changed in many ways, but I realize this is just the beginning. I walk every day at work on each of my breaks. I no longer snack at work like I used to. My lunch portions are healthy. I decreased my portions by nearly 70 percent and now I eat low carb, high protein foods and lots of veggies. I'm not nearly as tired as I used to be. I come home and go walking with my daughter. In the evenings, I clean up the kitchen, clean house or mow the lawn and I still have energy. I don't like to sit around like I used to do, but now I get moving as much as I can.

The biggest impact I have seen is that since I am less stressed. I respond in a healthier manner towards my family. In the past when I made changes, it was only in the physical. To really take the step to permanently change my lifestyle, I have to change my thoughts and mindset.[8] I have to be willing to crucify my flesh[9] and allow God to increase as I decrease.[10]

That's the big turning point for me — the big moment of change. I know that by being healthy in all aspects of my life, I am honoring God. More than that, I know I do not have to be afraid because God is my Protector.

Heather Tucker is a single mother, living in Southwest Missouri with her mother and daughter. She works in customer service. Her passion is to show the love of God to those who are broken and hurting.

ENDNOTES

1. Psalm 42:11 AMP
2. Jeremiah 29:11 NLT
3. Hebrews 12:1-2 NASB
4. Jeremiah 29:11 NIV
5. Jeremiah 29:12 NIV
6. Galatians 2:20 NIV
7. John 3:30 NIV
8. Romans 12:2 NIV
9. Galatians 2:20 NIV
10. John 3:30 NIV

CHAPTER 17

SUBTLE SHIFTS

What does it take to move a mountain? Making a monumental change seems like a daunting task. No matter what the mountain that needs to be moved looks like, it many times overwhelms and paralyzes us into a state of inactivity. It seems too difficult to climb, go around or tunnel through. The inactivity towards change makes the mountain loom larger and larger and larger.

Time has a way of enlarging the improbable to be utterly impossible. What looks big today, will look gigantic a year from now and monumental 10 years from now. The longer it sits without movement, the bigger it grows at least in the mind.

Without action, the mountain won't be removed, changed or eradicated overnight. For instance, if the mountain requires losing a large amount of weight it will take months, maybe even years. It won't happen with a short-term restriction in how a person eats or by purchasing a membership at a local gym.

What has to happen for health to be restored is a course correction, a subtle but meaningful shift. It starts in the mind with the way food is viewed. Food is fuel for the body to perform the tasks individuals have been assigned by God to carry out on this earth.

To lose weight, there must be a change of perspective on the purpose of food. Living solely for the purpose of eating will hasten an individual towards death. Eating to live is the purpose for which God provided food. This subtle play on words makes a big impact when implemented and adopted completely. This subtle shift has to be acted upon so a person no longer eats things based on how they look, smell or taste. The time for eating foods one craves must end.

The brain must be rewired to think about why one wants to eat certain things, what the body needs for optimal performance and how one will feel in the long-run, rather than providing the stomach's immediate pleasure. Up to this point, these subtle shifts are imperceptible because they are all occurring in the brain, redirecting thoughts so that eventually, feelings about food change. Then, behaviors follow suit because one has allowed God to begin the reprogramming process.

PERSISTENCE

Blasting away at the mountain and expecting it to crumble immediately doesn't really work. It takes persistent faith to move a mountain. If one has even the tiniest bit of faith he or she can say to the mountain, "Move and it will move."[1]

The time frame for mountain moving isn't described. We think it means immediately because that's just the type of society we live in. We want things done instantly. Speaking to the mountain, though, first takes convincing one's self that the mountain can be moved.

God already believes it. We don't have to convince Him. Most prayers for mountain-moving focus on convincing God the mountain needs to be moved. He has already told us how to move it. He gave us the key. It takes acting in faith for mountains to move. The shifts will be subtle as we begin to work consistently and persistently with faith and effort toward the goal of monumental change.

> God will give us sustenance and strength while we take steps forward so we can move the mountain.

There is not a recognizable difference to others when an extremely large person loses a few pounds. The one losing weight feels it, though. Clothes begin to fit differently. Chairs become easier to sit in. The seat in the car must be moved a little closer to the steering wheel.

It all happens because of the subtle mind shift juxtaposing words. "I am eating to live, not living to eat." It seemed like such a small thing at the time, but this time the brain believed it, adopted it and put it into action. This time it is real. This time it is backed up with faith and actions.

This time what seemed impossible is becoming possible because of trusting God's help on the journey. He won't move the mountain, but He gives sustenance and strength while we take steps forward so we can move the mountain.

These slight alternations in how we think will eventually result in astounding differences in our lives. One day we'll be looking through old pictures and we won't believe the change that has happened in just a few months or years.

We will go to our closet to get our favorite shirt from last year and realize it hangs on us now. We are excited to be able to give it away because we will never need it again. The new pair of jeans that was too small six months ago is now too big. Wearing them never even happened. A video of us sitting beside someone we always thought of as skinny reveals we are as small or smaller.

> God supported us when we put faith into action.

The mountain has moved when we weren't cognitively aware of the movement.

The ease of the movement cannot be attributed to our own self-effort, though. It was through the power of the Holy Spirit, the same power that raised Jesus from the dead.[2]

He supported us when we put faith into action. It was Him working through us, but we were cooperating with Him.

There's no better feeling than knowing we are obedient in joining with the mountain-moving God of the universe.

Subtle shifts, monumental changes and we are transformed.[3]

For Andrew Parker, the shift happened when he didn't realize it. Always thinking he couldn't lose weight, he began to realize he could. The idea changed his perceived lie into a truth and fueled a monumental change.

Please be aware as you read his story that when he is talking about his mother, I am the culprit.

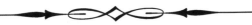

CHANGE STORY

ANDREW PARKER

I always thought of myself as the fat kid. I wasn't into sports, though I did like bike riding and going on hikes with my dad and sister. The whole idea of sports didn't appeal to me. I guess you might say I was more of a loner.

My uncle and cousin were into sports. We'd throw the football around some, but if I was outside I'd rather be on my scooter or bike. As a kid I discovered what I really liked most, though, was computers. I liked taking them apart and putting them back together. I also loved playing video games and watching TV. I remember once or twice staying up all night just so I would be up early enough to watch Beakman's World on Saturday morning.

> Though I didn't like being called the fat kid, I just figured it was who I was.

Given my lack of exercise and love of things that caused me to sit all day, it's no surprise that I gained weight early. Though I didn't like being called the fat kid, I just figured it was who I was. I never thought I could lose weight, so I never really tried.

I like people, but I do fine without them, too. Still, being overweight contributed to my lack of self-confidence.

In the 90s I discovered cargo pants. There is something about the function over fashion that I love, but the style was baggy cut and straight leg. It was always hard to find such pants in my size. I ended up wearing normal cargo pants that were larger than I needed from the big and tall men's shop. These pants were shaped like an inverted triangle with the point at the bottom of the leg expanding upward to a large waist. These were nothing like what I was looking for, but that's all I could find. A pair that fit at my waist would be tight on my legs and thighs. Larger pairs only afforded a bit wider leg and cinching down the waist on a larger pair was uncomfortable. Whatever I did, they fit horribly.

One of the best things about losing weight was just being able to buy pants from normal places like the mall and having them fit properly and feel comfortable. The kind of pants I liked in my size, 46-48, had to be bought online. Now, I am in a size 36-38 pants and L or XL shirts. Before, I was wearing a 3X shirt.

FOOD GALORE

After high school, I went to college part-time and worked part-time. I was still living at home. My mother was quite large at the time and there were always desserts, any kind of food and snacks galore to eat. My family joked about me being the garbage disposal. Leftovers did not have to be thrown away when I was around because I'd finish them off. Mom would say, "Eat the last of those brownies. Finish off those last two hamburgers." And so being a good kid, I'd do it.

I never really saw food as a substitute for anything. I just ate without thinking about it. It never crossed my mind that I might be able to lose weight. I just thought it was my lot in life to be overweight.

In 2012, I got the opportunity to train as an Apple® service technician. The company owned a store in Colorado and needed a service manager there right away. I had a week to pack and be there. Initially after arriving, I stayed with the manager. Because I was in someone else's home, I didn't feel I had free access to their food. Whatever I ate was what I bought or I ate at local restaurants. In other words, there was not an unlimited supply of food like there was at home.

Being active was infectious.

I found I didn't miss all the food. I found food wasn't that important. I had too many other things on my mind what with being in a new place with new people, being away from my family and friends and trying to decide if I wanted to stay in this line of work. With my busy schedule and all the fun things to do in town, I didn't focus on food.

Glenwood Springs, CO, is a very active community and being active was infectious. People were active just because it's fun. It wasn't necessarily because they felt they needed to be thinner or to punish themselves for eating too much. The town is small, but the downtown area, where the store was located, is bustling with activity. It made more sense to walk places because I had to park a distance from the store. Going to get the car four blocks away to go somewhere three blocks away and then probably not finding a place to park didn't make any sense. So anywhere I went downtown I would just walk.

Growing up in the suburbs this was a novel concept to me. I could be in one place, say work, and walk to another, say a restaurant for lunch, without ever having to use a car. When I did eat out, I only ate at local restaurants that weren't fast food chains, to sample local cuisine. Most served primarily organic food and lean meat, like buffalo burgers for example.

Biking is big in Colorado, especially in Glenwood Springs. As a matter of fact, one is considered kind of weird if he or she doesn't ride a bike. So in keeping with my newfound interest in alternative transportation styles, I became a regular bike rider. When I moved out of the boss's apartment, I made sure to find a place that was accessible to town by foot or bike. I started biking to work. I also biked to places like to the grocery store and carried my purchases home in my backpack.

One morning I woke up to get ready for work. The room I was staying in had a full-length mirror on the wall. I noticed I looked thinner and my pants were looser. I figured I was fooling myself somehow. I couldn't be losing weight. However, every day I looked at the mirror and I kept looking thinner.

I bought a scale to verify whether it was true. I had lost weight. It might have been just 10 pounds or so then, but at the time I thought it was impossible for me to lose weight. I figured I could maintain and not get fatter if I wanted to, but lose? Impossible.

MOMENT OF CHANGE

This was my moment of change. I decided that all the things I was doing by accident, I would do on purpose. I would run with it and help out the process. I didn't know I could start losing weight again if I stopped because it had never happened before. So I figured I might as well lose as much as possible.

I stopped eating at any major fast food chains. I stayed away from high fructose corn syrup. I started being more active.

I was busy and didn't have much time to eat, so that could have contributed as well. I was eating at around 2 and 9 p.m. I normally stay up late anyway, so eating supper late meant I wasn't snacking constantly.

Something I'd always wanted to do was buy some Kangoo Jumps. These are sort of like boots with springs on the bottom. They help you run faster and jump higher. I had wanted to buy a pair for some time, but I was over the weight limit. By now my weight had gone from 275 to under 250, which was below the limit, and I could buy a pair.

EXERCISE CAN BE FUN

Kangoo Jumps are kind of expensive, but seeing this as my chance to really lose some weight, I decided to just go ahead and buy a pair to reward myself. I figured it would be a good way to get myself to exercise more because it looked fun. It was summer and the perfect time to start.

I'd Kangoo Jump around town when I could find the time, mostly at night after work or on weekends. The company's website says Kangoo Jumping equates to intense cardio and I was doing it in the thin mountain air. This definitely jump-started my weight loss. At one point I was featured in a local newspaper article calling me the seven-foot tall man. I'm only about six feet tall, but the Kangoo Jumps made me seem that tall.

I've learned exercise can be fun. It doesn't have to be a mean gym teacher yelling at me. I can choose to have fun in my own way. Biking is something I love to do. I'm now back in Columbia and although there are some great biking trails, there is really no way to go from where I live on a bike without going on roads that aren't designed for bike traffic.

So I park in a grocery store parking lot and ride my bike from there to the places I want to go. Why? Because I can and it's fun. Yes, it helps keep my weight under control, but more than that I really enjoy it.

I used to drink sugary sodas all the time because it just seemed to be what we drank with meals in my family. Now, I drink mainly water. I drink cold filtered or purified water and take it with me wherever I go, especially on long bike rides. I will drink a soda every once in awhile. When I do drink soda I make sure it's a good quality gourmet or organic soda. I appreciate it more that way than when I'm drinking it like water.

In sixth grade I had stopped drinking caffeinated sodas. I saw caffeine as a drug. Eliminating caffeine sodas mostly left me with just a lemon lime soda, which can get old quickly. Limiting soda was an easy step for me to make.

MY FOOD GAME

I do eat sugar, but I keep the amount of times I indulge to a minimum. I try to keep it down to at most once a day. That way I have to be picky about when I want it. Do I want to eat sugary cereal for breakfast, have a soda in the evening, or some ice cream after dinner? Some days I don't do any of these.

Sometimes I want to eat a certain sugary food and I tell myself, "Okay, fine, you can have it, but just wait until tomorrow. If you still want it, then you can have it." And sometimes tomorrow comes and I don't want it. Other times I do this every day for like a week and I still want it, so I go ahead and have it.

In the meantime, I've managed to trick myself into not indulging in sweets for a week. Another thing I've learned, if I start to want the same thing over and over again, I stop eating it altogether for a time.

I treat it as a game. Let's see how long Andrew can go without sweets. That way there's less stress involved. There is no personal integrity at stake and I don't feel like I'm putting harsh restrictions on myself because I can stop anytime I want. The operable part of this is that I can stop, yet I understand that others cannot and so they need to not indulge at all.

> When I became consistent with eating healthier and moving more, losing weight got eaiser.

One thing I have learned that may be beneficial to people trying to lose weight is that fat has momentum, just as an object that is in motion tends to stay in motion and an object at rest tends to stay at rest, the same applies to losing weight.

The first couple of pounds seemed to be the hardest to lose. When I became consistent with eating healthier and moving more, losing weight got easier. It's like when I have to push my car when it breaks down. Just getting it to move at all is the hardest part, but when it starts rolling it becomes much easier.

Consistency is the key. Before I would do active things like going on bike rides and try to eat a bit healthier every once in a blue moon, but I never kept at it long enough to get my weight to move. It's like my body was saying, "Hold on. This is just a false alarm. Everything is going back to normal soon."

It wasn't until my eating and excercise habits had consistently changed that my body thought, "Okay, well I guess he does mean it this time. Might as well make some changes."

> After losing 50 pounds, I am more self-confident and assured I am doing all that I can to be the best I can be.

With the list of largely sedentary things I still love to do and the fact the types of food I like to eat have not changed, such as pizza, hamburgers, etc., and the fact that I just turned 30 this year, I am concerned about gaining weight. However, I have changed the way I look at food and myself.

In addition, I have learned a few things. Soda is not water. I don't have to have sweets all the time. Being active can be fun and even beneficial to my emotional well being. I have also started down a road of discovering abilities I did not know I had. Chief of these is that I do have the capacity to lose weight. Knowing that, I feel a responsibility to keep tabs on what I eat.

Today, I just enjoy living in a body that is more fit and healthy. After losing 50 pounds, I am more self-confident and assured I am doing all that I can to be the best I can be.

I'm growing up and realizing I can take control of my life, my body and my career. I can be the man of God He called me to be.

I do not have to remain the fat kid. He left the room a long time ago.

Andrew Parker lives in Columbia Mo, where he is an independent Apple® and Windows Computer Technician. Besides biking, hiking and computer games, his other loves are a 1993 Honda Civic and two Birman Cats, Harley and Fluff.

ENDNOTES

1. Matthew 17:20 NIV
2. Romans 8:11 NIV
3. Romans 12:1-2 NLT

SWEET CHANGE

NINE THINGS MINUS SUGAR

'm addicted to sugar. How do I stop? It's a question I'm asked a lot. When I was struggling with this addiction all I wanted was to follow a plan, like a recipe. I wanted to follow it exactly so I would get a perfect outcome.

The ingredients for beating sugar addiction, however, are not exact. The only thing I'm sure of is that processed sugar is not one of the ingredients. For a processed sugar addict, that is like a hard blow to the mid-section. The one thing an addict never wants to surrender is the source of their addiction.

> An addict never wants to surrender the source of their addiction.

However, it is the one thing that must be given up. I will try to explain the process I went through, but to put it in a step-by-step plan is not so easy. Some steps seem to wander in and out of each other blurring the lines.

Acceptance — Admitting "I have a problem," is the first step. For years I accepted I had a problem. I was super morbidly obese. That was one thing I couldn't ignore. I tried and tried and tried to fix it by myself. After all, I was pretty good at fixing other problems. I ran a household, a business and a ministry. I had a husband, two children and two foster children. I wasn't sure why I couldn't fix my issue with extreme weight gain so I could continue to hang on to everything I thought I couldn't live without.

> Giving up processed sugar sounded impossible. I figured there must be an easier way.

Realization — An important ingredient to beating sugar addiction is the realization there is an answer. The answer didn't sound appealing when I first heard about it. Actually, it was God who revealed the plan to me. At the time giving up processed sugar sounded impossible. I figured surely there must be an easier way.

Through the years, God continued to reveal the same plan to me when I would get frustrated with my situation. It took over three decades for me to come to the end of my rope. After exhausting every other possibility, I finally realized the only way to start really living was to stop eating sugar.

Surrender — When it was time to surrender sugar I understood one very big thing. I had been going to sugar instead of to God. Sugar had been my resource for anesthetizing any emotion. To undo it, I had to let go of emotional attachments to people and things from my past.

I had to reach towards the only One who had always been there to support me. When I reached up to Him, He reached down to me. I had to understand was that surrender meant giving up what I was addicted to for the rest of my life.

The actual moment of surrender didn't come with bells and whistles, but with just letting go. I let go of sugar to take hold of the hand of the One who had been there all along.

Repentance — I had been walking one way towards a very unhealthy life. I knew the direction I needed to go. I thought of all the ways through the years I'd tried to get there. I had taken many circuitous routes that seemed to only take me farther away from my destination. Now, I was faced with the truth. To get to health, I had to turn around and go in the opposite direction.

I could not carry extra supplies for a relapse. I had to lay everything down. It was an all or nothing proposition. I had been going the wrong way. I admitted my failure. I didn't just say I was sorry. I repented once and for all. I turned around and began the journey towards health. I did not look back for to look back would mean I would again turn into a pillar of sugar.

> To get to health, I had to turn around and go in the opposite direction. I did not look back for to look back would mean I would again turn into a pillar of sugar.

Obedience — Walking out the journey is where many get scared and run back to the comfort zone of addiction they've always relied on. To walk in obedience, there has to be a Higher Power to which obedience is given. For me that Higher Power is God. He is the One who beckoned me on this journey for decades. He is the One to whom I run to now in obedience.

Walking in obedience ties the hands of the supposed strong man who calls to me in times when I have always run to sugar. I stand in the power of God, face the accuser and say, "No, I am a child of obedience. I will no longer listen to you." When I say this by my lifestyle, he knows he has lost and after some time of continuing to badger he will go bother someone else.

Momentum — Grace is the operational power of God that brings momentum to my journey. I begin with trepidation and a quiet whisper in my heart telling me, "No, this is the way, walk here."[1]

As I walk, I soon begin to pick up speed and before I know it I am running with the wind of grace at my back, almost as if it is a race. My Author is always clearly in sight urging me on.[2]

> The transformation I desire is a journey from glory to glory to become more like the Master.

There is no possibility of turning back now, knowing what He endured so I can run this race. I have surrendered it all to Him and I will not turn back. The momentum is strong and yet there are days I feel so weak.[3] He runs before me so I know exactly where to go. Because of His direction I don't fall or falter, but run boldly with courage.[4]

Transformation — The transformation I desire is a journey from glory to glory[5] to become more and more like the Master. I look at my body after five years of walking this journey and I know a transformation is taking place. I continue to make decisions not to give in to everything the world tells me.

My mind is continually renewed and changed. Which decisions come first? Which are decisions learned along the journey? I know not. I only know I continue to make the choices necessary for the transformation to continue.[6]

Victory — I am victorious in many aspects. Yet, I do not assume I have won the victory for to do so would be to let my guard down. I still keep my eyes ever on my Author and Guide. Victory comes only through Christ.

For years I knew I needed a victory that could only come through deliverance.[7] I cried out to have the chains that bound me broken. What I didn't understand was I had placed myself in the chains. Only I had the key to set myself free.

Victory comes in surrender. When I hold on to the things I crave, the things I think I can't live without, I

> The same power that raised Christ from the dead is raising me from the death trap I placed myself in.

can never be free. There is only one place complete victory is found. It is in the One who overcame all of earth's temptations. The same power that raised Christ from the dead[8] is raising me up from the death trap I placed myself in.

The victory comes only by placing everything at the feet of Jesus and keeping it there. There can be nothing held back. There can be nothing retrieved. For years, I thought I was hiding my addiction from Him. I'd say I surrendered it, but I hadn't. I hadn't given it totally to Him. He knew it because He knew my heart.

The moment my heart was right, though, I appropriated the operational power found in grace. I was catapulted forward. I felt it as a blast of love, a door of hope flung wide open.

Freedom — When along the journey did it happen that I surrendered totally? I know it happened to begin the journey, but it also happens as I continue to daily find myself with my face on the floor before Him, crying out for His strength.

> I know I have found freedom from the things I have been bound to all my life. Total surrender. Total victory. Total freedom.

He strengthens me because my heart is now totally His.[9] And I know I have found freedom from the things I have been bound to all my life. Total surrender. Total victory. Total freedom.

Can I turn back and pick it all back up again? Yes, at any moment because He has given me free will. I have a choice. I can choose bondage or I can choose freedom. I will never go back because nothing tastes as good as freedom feels. Nothing.

Mindy Nave is in the beginning stages of her sugar-free journey. She is ready for the ride of her life. She is determined her motto will be, "no turning back."

CHANGE STORY
MINDY NAVE

On my 37th birthday, I finally accepted the best gift I've ever been given — life. I didn't realize it, but I was dying a slow death from my favorite drug — sugar. It was making me sick in every way. My body. My spirit. My soul.

My life was slipping away from me and I felt powerless to stop it. What I thought was helping me feel in control was actually causing me to lose control. I knew the Heavenly Father was asking me to let it go and surrender it to Him. I knew He wanted me to trust that He could and would help me, but I didn't know if that was possible.

> What I thought was helping me be in control was causing me to lose control.

I wanted to believe I could hold on to it and still stay in control, but I had proven to myself in the past that it's just too addictive to me. One bite, one drink, one taste and I would be sucked in and feel compelled to have more, my hunger for it ever increasing.

After the pleasure quickly dissipated, I would find myself back in reality. I felt tired and sick. Sick and tired. I felt guilty and ashamed. I felt trapped. I felt powerless to my addiction.

I had dabbled in giving it up before, but to give it up totally? That felt impossible. However, after celebrating one more birthday with sugary treats, I surrendered it forever — my lover, my friend, my drug of choice — sugar.

I made my decision. I decided to finally stand up and say "no" to this trap from my enemy. He has been trying to steal, kill and destroy me[10] and I was allowing him to do it. With that last bite of brownie, I said "Good-bye forever" to sugar and all the false feelings of security and comfort it had given me for so long.

> Sugar plays a huge role in whether or not I will be successful in losing weight.

This new journey without sugar is not going to be easy. This is one of the hardest things I've ever done. I know in my own strength I can't do it, but I know with the Father's help, I can. I am weak, but He is strong.[11]

My husband and I started getting interested in learning about better health a few years ago. Over time, I've heard a lot about the addictive nature of sugar. However, it was when I tried to give it up, but felt drawn to it like a magnet that I discovered just how addictive it truly was. Once I realized how much damage it was doing to my body, soul and spirit, I knew the Father was asking me to surrender it.

Weight loss definitely plays a role in my decision. I have battled with my weight since my early 20s. I know now that sugar plays a huge role in whether or not I will be successful in losing weight. Now, that I have finally let it go, I feel armed and ready to lose 30 pounds or more and keep my weight stable.

Obesity is common in my family. When I reached 245 pounds, I knew something had to change. Although I was an emotional eater in my teenage years, I was able to maintain a size 8-10 until I went to college. I then gained the typical "freshman 15" and ended up dropping out after one semester when I became employed at an office job.

I got married and the weight began to pile on. My emotional eating dramatically increased when it became evident I was struggling with infertility. Within five years, I had put on 100 pounds. I eventually became pregnant and used that as an excuse to continue to eat carelessly.

Seven months after our son was born, my world fell apart when I found myself a single mom. Then, two weeks later, I discovered I was pregnant with our second son. I realized I would be going through this pregnancy alone. I fell into a dark time and continued to overeat and put on more weight than necessary.

Because of my addiction to sugar and a continued struggle with emotional eating, I have gone up and down with my weight.

After my son was born, the divorce was final and I felt a door close on my past. At that point, I was ready for a new beginning. I began to focus on losing weight and feeling better about myself.

Over a period of about five months, I lost 75 pounds and felt great at a weight of 170 pounds. I was in a new relationship and got married. Since that time, I have given birth to two girls and now have four precious children.

I've managed to stay under 200 pounds, but because of my addiction to sugar and a continued struggle with emotional eating, I have gone up and down with my weight. I feel confident that letting go of sugar forever is going to have a big impact on my success in losing the weight I need to lose and keeping it off for good.

I love to ride my bicycle and plan to get into a regular routine of exercising with workout videos at home. I feel my best when I'm taking care of my body. I know this will make me a healthier and happier person. I want to leave a legacy of good health for my children. It's important to me that they see me making good choices that will affect our whole family. Giving up sugar for good was one of the most difficult, but most powerful choices I could make.

Surrendering to Him and trusting Him to help me overcome sugar addiction has changed me.

When I made it through my first day without sugar, I must say, I felt different — not so much physically yet, but emotionally. It felt as if in the past I had been wrestling with the Heavenly Father. I knew in my heart He was asking me to give up sugar, but it felt impossible.

I was absolutely miserable in my rebellion. I was double-minded. Like the Bible says, "Being double-minded man (or woman) unstable in all his (or her) ways."[12] That's exactly the truth.

I know now without a doubt that there is absolutely no replacement for the King of kings. He is jealous for me.

He doesn't want me to have idols in my life. He wants and deserves to have first place in my heart. While I was allowing my addiction to control my life, I wasn't able to live completely for Him.

My life is different now. Surrendering to Him and trusting Him to help me overcome this sugar addiction has changed me. I feel so much more peace in my heart now. I'm a better wife and a better mom because I'm not wrestling with the Heavenly Father or myself anymore. Wrestling will wear a person out in every way.

The miserable feeling that comes with disobedience went away as soon as I let go of my addiction and truly surrendered it to Him. I have been given a second chance at a healthy life. I have clarity about what I need to do. I am on a journey towards a life lived in the freedom that my relationship with the Messiah brings.

ANTICIPATING THE FUTURE

For me, not eating processed sugar changes things tremendously. It means saying no to temptation every day for the rest of my life. It means I have to have a plan in place for all the situations that could lead to failure, such as family dinners, birthday parties, potlucks and social situations. It means I will sometimes feel alone, especially when I'm the only one not eating certain foods. It means everything is changing when it comes to the foods I buy and eat.

Since obesity, diabetes and heart disease run in my family, I want to do whatever I can to stay free of them. For me, sugar is a guaranteed ticket to poor health. I will not be getting back on that train. Ever.

I never want to go back to eating sugar again. I don't want to be that woman anymore — the one who felt powerless and incapable of being free. I don't want to be the mom I was before — irritable and unkind because of the sugar coursing through my veins, chemically altering my behavior and my moods.

> Sugar is my nemesis and I plan to stay as far away from it as possible.

I have a calling on my life to help hurting people and take them into a deeper relationship with the Father through worship music. I know that it will only happen to the degree that I'm willing to surrender things standing between Him and me.

Sugar is my nemesis and I plan to stay as far away from it as possible.

I believe. I surrender. I trust. It is finished. Life and health are waiting for me. I'm taking off in that direction. I surrender completely to Him.

No turning back.

Mindy Nave is a wife and homeschooling mom of four and lives in Boonville, MO. As a speaker, Mindy shares her story to encourage others to find the freedom available through the Savior. A worship leader, singer and keyboard player, you can find her on YouTube channel mindysue77.

ENDNOTES

1. Isaiah 30:21 NIV
2. Hebrews 12:1-2 NIV
3. Hebrews 12:12, 2 Corinthians 12:9-10 NIV
4. Hebrews 12:13 NIV
5. 2 Corinthians 3:17-18 NIV
6. Romans 12:2 NIV
7. Romans 7:24-25 NIV
8. Romans 8:11 NIV
9. Chronicles 16:9 NIV
10. John 10:10 NIV
11. 2 Corinthians 12:10 NIV
12. James 1:8 NASB

SWEET CHANGE

CHAPTER 19

AMAZING DESTINY

To go on a change journey of any kind is a rather scary, but totally exhilarating proposition. To tell you the truth, I didn't know what I was getting myself into. For one time in my life, I didn't overthink it. Realizing I was an addict, only with sugar, was the major turning point. That realization really hit me hard.

Many people who don't have an issue with weight just assume every person who is extremely overweight is lazy, unintelligent and has no self-control. This is not true. However, I had bought into this lie myself thinking that if I would just try harder I could overcome this issue.

GRACE AND WORKS

Understanding the issue was way bigger than something I could control was the best thing that ever happened to me. I had what some might call a do-it-yourself faith. I certainly knew I was saved by grace, but I also thought I had to demonstrate I was saved by doing good works. This whole "doing" part of faith was constantly on my mind.

Towards the end of her life, my grandmother would ask me that question when I would read her Revelation 21, which is the description of heaven. And even though it says right there at the end of that chapter, that only whose names are in Book of Life will enter heaven,[1] Grandma would still ask. "But have I done enough to get in?"

> Yes, Jesus loves me and I love Him.

I'd tell her again how it's not about how much we've done, but that we have trusted and believed completely in the One who loves us, died for us and rose again victorious so that we could go to heaven if we only believe in Him. Then, she'd remember Him and smile and say, "Yes, Jesus loves me and I love Him."

After my grandfather had died, Grandma began her volunteer career. She volunteered at the hospital, at a thrift store, for her church, with her club and was always available to help those in need.

She was demonstrating her faith by her actions. It was part of who she was. She didn't do it because she had to, but at end of her life she wondered, does God keep score? Could it be He says to us, "Sorry, you are one volunteer job short of getting in to heaven. You missed it by this much."

There is a difference between being created to do positive things and feeling like we have to do them to prove we are saved or to prove to God we are good enough to make it into heaven. No one is good enough. That's why Jesus' sacrifice was so important. He pays our entrance fee into heaven if we just put all our trust in Him.

"We have become His poetry, a recreated people that will fulfill the destiny He has given each of us, for we are joined to Jesus, the Anointed One. Even before we were born, God planned in advance our destiny and the good works we would do to fulfill it."[2]

I love the way The Passion Translation helps us understand that when we accept Christ we are recreated so that we get to fulfill His destiny for our lives. It's not about what we should do, but what we get to do.

God has this amazing destiny already planned out for us. We get to do good stuff, but only if we're free, only if we're no longer in bondage and love some things more than God. To me that's what addiction is — it's loving something more than I love God.

> When we accept Christ, we are recreated so that we get to fulfill His destiny for our lives.

We can be addicted to many things. After writing *Sweet Grace*, a worship pastor emailed me. He told me he related to my story, however his addiction was not food, but pornography. I told him surrendering, totally giving it up to God, was the only way to freedom. His last email to me said, "I can only hope, I can find the freedom you have found in Christ." It felt very much like his hope was just wishful thinking because there was no surrender attached to it.

To find freedom from our bondages we have to stand firm against them. "It is for freedom that Christ has set us free. Stand firm, then, and do not let yourselves be burdened again by a yoke of slavery."[3]

The crux of this is very much tied up with our destiny. Only those who have allowed God to totally recreate every part of them are really free. And only those who are really free can tap into the destiny God has already planned for them.

GOD HAS GREATER FOR YOU

Years ago, I read *Experiencing God* by Henry Blackaby. I was especially struck by one story he told about deciding his son was old enough for a bicycle for his birthday. He went out and bought a blue Schwinn bike and hid it in the garage. Then his job was to convince his son he needed exactly that. It wasn't long before his son decided what he really wanted for his birthday was a blue Schwinn bicycle.

Blackaby says, "The bike was already in the garage. I just had to convince him to ask for it. He asked for it, and he got it." He points out that the same thing happens with us and Holy Spirit. The Holy Spirit's job is to get us to want what He already has for us.

"What will happen when you ask for things God already want to give or do?" Blackaby says. "You will always receive it."

God wants the best for us, but before He can make it available for us we have to be in the mode to receive it. He will not give us a bicycle that we cannot ride because of a lifestyle issue. He will not immediately help us reach a destiny when we are not ready for it.

For years I wanted to write a book. The book God had waiting in the garage for me to write, was my own story of deliverance from sugar addiction. Had I not gone on the journey I did, I would have never taken what I see now was the first step towards my true destiny, the thing He planned in advance for me to do before I was even born.

Had I remained entrenched in bondage and addiction, chained in cell for which I already had the key, I would most likely not be alive today. That would have been a choice of my own making.

Change is not easy, but it is worth everything, even our very lives. It is the key to walking in the victory Jesus brings. We can be Christians and still live in bondage, never stepping into the greater things God has stored for us in His monumental warehouse.

> Change is not easy, but it is worth everything, even our very lives. It is the key to walking in the victory Jesus brings.

We cry out for His blessings, but are we willing to go through the continual changes it takes for us to step into the things He already has for us? We are a recreated people, however we continually want to crawl out of the chrysalis and circumvent the process of change.

"Therefore, if anyone is in Christ, he is a new creation; old things have passed away; behold, all things have become new."[4] Most of us think this is an automatic new creation. We do receive all the tools we need to become new when we accept Christ. Some of us, though, pick up new things that put us into bondage along the way. Change needs to be ongoing as we are being transformed into His image from glory to glory.[5]

He has this over the top destiny in store for us. It's just waiting. He has it all planned. It was planned before we were born. We probably only know the tip of the iceberg.

> He has this over-the-top destiny in store for us. He has it all planned.

"Never doubt God's mighty power to work in you and accomplish all of this. He will achieve infinitely more than your greatest request, your most unbelievable dream, and exceed your wildest imagination. He will outdo them all for His miraculous power constantly energizes you."[6]

I tapped into this miraculous power when I surrendered the thing I had withheld from God for years — my addiction to processed sugar. I have begun to understand the greater things He has in store for me and every believer when we will admit their weakness and accept His strength[7] for our lives.

ENDNOTES

1. Revelation 21:27 NIV
2. Ephesians 2:10 TPT
3. Galatians 5:1 NIV
4. 2 Corinthians 5:17 NKJV
5. 2 Corinthians 3:18 NKJV
6. Ephesians 3:20 TPT
7. 2 Corinthians 12:9-10 NLT

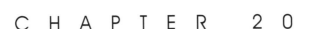

CHAPTER 20

FINAL NOTE

The way to know if you've had a moment of change is what happens after you make the decision. There is the moment of decision, but there were many other moments leading up to the moment of change and many to come after.

What we must wrap our brains around is that success comes only when we are committed to a total lifestyle change. Our moments after the change can be nothing like the moments before. We must step out of what has become a comfortable routine and start on a journey that WILL change our lives.

For me that had to include a mentor, an accountability group and an intentional connection with God. It also included a team of doctors and specialists, a fitness trainer, regular time in the pool, learning to cook differently and a great plan called stop-start.

CHANGE WORK

I began the real change work on this journey five years ago. Last year when I was writing my memoir, *Sweet Grace*, I experienced God as Provider. When I didn't know how to do something, I would simply pray and He would lead me to the answer. I experienced the same with this book. He's always a step ahead of me. He always has the resources I need to take the next step.

After I published *Sweet Grace,* my life started exploding in a good way. I got requests to speak, do radio and TV interviews and lead workshops. These things were never on my radar.

God has taken me on an amazing journey and has shown me I am self-sufficient through Christ's sufficiency.[1] If He leads me to do something, He will provide the resources I need to do it.

FAITH

Today, I live not knowing what the next major event will be. I call it simply living not knowing. Knowing God knows is enough for me. There are goals and plans I have in place, but I always know He can interrupt them anytime He chooses because the life I live is not my own. It is for His glory.[2]

We control our lives out of fear. When we really believe we can trust God for every detail, we will begin to let go of the need to control.

When my life began going fast and furious last year, my time couldn't be stretched any further, so I had to delegate things to others. I realized very quickly life's ride is much smoother when I give the wheel over to God. After all, He's the only One who can get me where I need to go.

So I live by faith. I live not knowing what is coming next. Though I never thought it would be true of me, I love it. The sense of being overwhelmed has been replaced with peace, focus and direction. I don't have to worry about how to do the next step. He's already got it planned. My job is to rest in Him, soak in His presence, let go of fear, take His hand and step out.

I've learned I can operate in faith on a day-to-day basis because I know there is substance to the firm hope I have. God's promises are not some nebulous wishes in my brain. They are real because He is real. I can point to the many times He's led me through the years. I know His promises have substance.[3] There's peace in hope backed by God's power. I can't touch or see God, but I have evidence[4] of how He has worked in my life and in the lives of many others. I know He is real so I can place my faith solidly in Him.

GRACE

Sometimes taking a step of faith feels risky. The risk is not in who God is, but in who I am and my ability to follow what I feel He's leading me to do. When I take that step of faith, though, I fall right into the arms of grace.

He catches me and sets my feet back on the path, if they've strayed. Maybe He just points me in the right direction if I've wandered off the path.[5] Most of the time, He buoys me up and propels me forward on the path.

I couldn't lose weight, write a book, publish a book, speak, coach, write a second book until I believed God was calling me to do it and I stepped out. At the point of stepping out is where grace kicks in. It's not there until I step out. One second before,

I couldn't do it. When I step out, before my foot hits the ground His grace is there providing the power for the task.

It's very true in every aspect, but I have to say it's even more true on this weight loss journey. God knows us. He knows when we're being honest about our surrender to Him. When He knew I'd experienced that shift, that moment of change, He brought every one of His resources to bear in my life.

WHAT'S NEXT?

What many people need is just someone to walk the journey with them. One doesn't have to be an expert to lead a group. Join several others and read this book together. If you've not read *Sweet Grace*, do that and complete the *Sweet Grace Study Guide* together. If you are honest with yourself and the group and do the work, with God's strength you can change. You can.

If you need my help, the best way to connect with me on this weight loss process is through the Sweet Change Weight Loss Coaching and Accountability Group. Those willing to invest in themselves realize this is for their lives. They will put their entire heart and soul into the change process. They will listen to the videos, do the action steps, ask questions, post their homework, implement the stop-start process and stop making excuses, all in a safe, confidential environment.

The process works to the extent each individual is willing to do the work. My mentor has said to me many times, "I can't want this for you more than you want it for yourself." I've seen that in Sweet Change Group. Those who want it, really want it, will not let anything stop them. Many are making great strides and having breakthroughs

Now it's time for you to make a decision. Is it time for you to take the next step to experience your breakthrough? Is it time for you to get real about your journey? Is it time for you to change your life and lose the weight you've always wanted to lose by focusing on your total being — body, soul and spirit?

HOW BADLY DO YOU WANT IT?

Let me ask you this: how badly do you want to lose the weight? How badly do you want to fit into that pair of jeans, cute top, nice dress or even, your wedding dress? You have dreams and goals, but how badly do you want to achieve them? You can do this, if you want to.

I want it for you, but I know I can't want it for you more than you want it for yourself. I can't motivate you to lose weight. Here's what I can do. I can give you guidance, tell you how to do this, what to release, how to get your mind in shape for the journey, how to throw aside unwanted baggage, how to accept God's help to get you to your next step. I can tell you, but you have to want it. The want you must provide. And I'm telling you, your want has to be big to get you to the place you want to be.

I couldn't have lost the amount of weight I lost without what Russ calls others, another and the Other. I had a weight loss group I went to, led by Russ. Both of these pointed me to the process of change. My Lord and Savior sealed the deal by calling to remembrance the lessons I learned in my group.

When I began my journey I had a hard time finding a group to do exactly what this group did for me — supporting me out of my food addiction and into freedom. I feel God dropped in my heart to start Sweet Change Weight Loss Coaching and Accountability Group as an online experience so those from all regions of the United States and all over the world can participate.

We currently have individuals from three foreign countries, as well many parts of the United States, even the state of Alaska. God is doing something phenomenal with this group and I'm inviting you to be a part. As one woman put it, "If I cut out going through fast food every day, I will save more than enough to join the group."

Joining Sweet Change and really participating will transform your life. I'm willing to be your coach and mentor. For the group to work for you, you must be willing to do the work. Intentional choices, intentional efforts pay off with intentional change.

Now, go to http://teresashieldsparker.com/sweet-change/ to discover the program details and sign up. You can be on your way to a sweet change today.

ENDNOTES

1. Philippians 4:13 AMP
2. 1 Corinthians 6:20 NASB
3. Hebrews 11:1 NKJV
4. ibid.
5. Isaiah 30:21 NIV

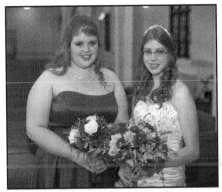

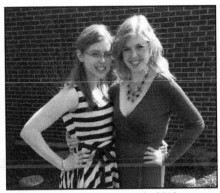

Lindsey Summers, left, with her sister, Brittany Lange in 2012.

Lindsey, right, with Brittany in 2013.

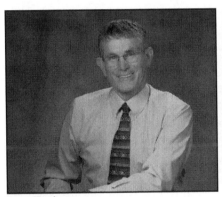

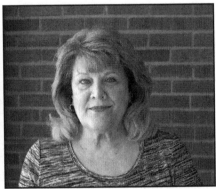

Russ Hardesty

Pam Leverett

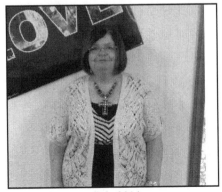

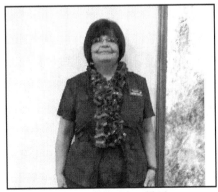

Rhonda Burrows, July 2014

Rhonda Burrows, December 2014

PHOTO PAGES

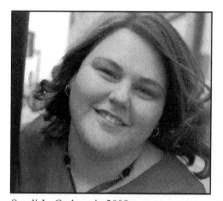

Sundi Jo Graham in 2008.

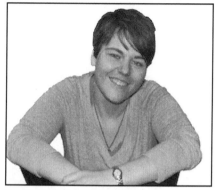

Sundi Jo, 145 pounds lighter.

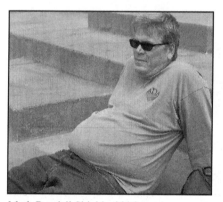

Mark Randall Shields, 2005.

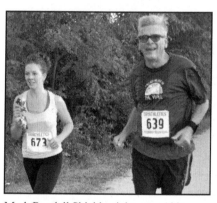

Mark Randall Shields, right, over 100 pounds lighter and running a half marathon.

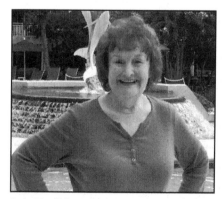

Judy English

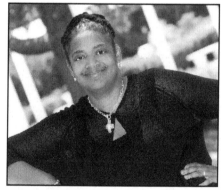

Aida Ingram

PHOTO PAGES

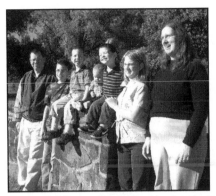

Anastacia Maness didn't like this picture of her with her family in 2012.

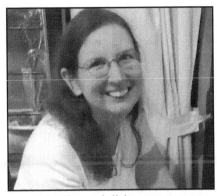

Anastacia, 53 pounds lighter.

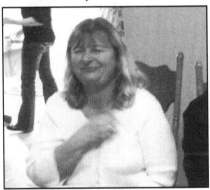

People used to have to sneak to take pictures of Kimberly Weger.

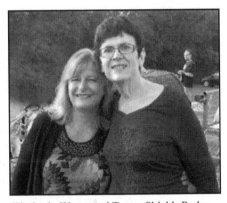

Kimberly Weger and Teresa Shields Parker in 2014. Kim is 50 pounds lighter.

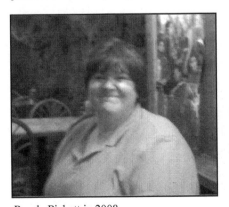

Ronda Pickett in 2008.

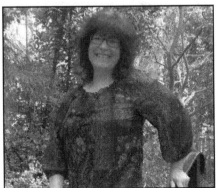

Ronda Pickett Waltman, 109 pounds lighter.

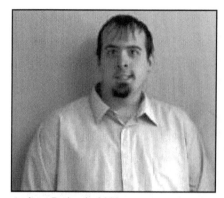

Andrew Parker in 2008.

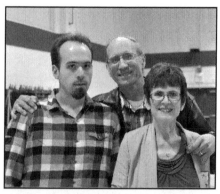

Andrew Parker in 2013 with Roy and Teresa Parker. He has lost 50 pounds.

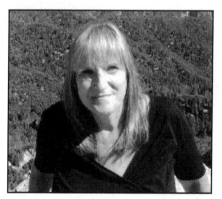

Nora Ann Treguboff Saggese

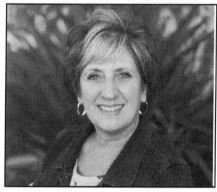

Donna Falcioni Barr

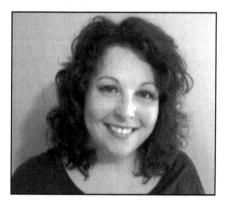

Heather Tucker

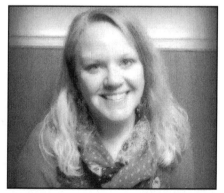

Mindy Nave

TERESA SHIELDS PARKER
BEFORE AND AFTER PHOTOS

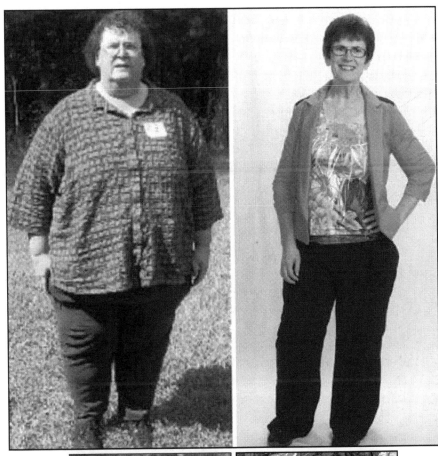

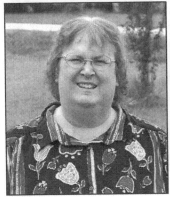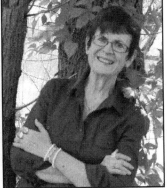

What's next?

SWEET CHANGE

WEIGHT LOSS COACHING & ACCOUNTABILITY GROUP

JOIN SWEET CHANGE WEIGHT LOSS COACHING GROUP for support, encouragement, weekly videos, action steps, accountability, monthly live call, mentorship, interaction with Teresa Shields Parker, 24/7 group access — all centered around the total approach to weight loss, becoming free and healthy — body, soul and spirit. For more information and testimonials from members go to: http://teresashieldsparker.com/sweet-change/

TAKE THE VIDEO COURSE SWEET CHANGE 101: Seven Keys for the Weight Loss Journey. Includes videos on the seven keys, along with study guides and action steps. Recommended before joining Sweet Change Group. Go to http://teresashieldsparker.com/sweet-change-101/. Other video short courses are on the web site.

SUBSCRIBE to Teresa's website for ongoing articles and updates at http://teresashieldsparker.com.

LIKE US ON FACEBOOK: http://www.facebook.com/ TeresaShieldsParker.

FOLLOW US ON TWITTER. https://twitter.com/ TreeParker

FOLLOW US ON PINTEREST: http://www. pinterest.com/treeparker/

SWEET GRACE

"Sweet Grace: How I Lost 250 Pounds and Stopped Trying To Earn God's Favor" is Teresa Shields Parker's weight loss memoir. Read the remarkable story of how she lost 250 pounds. Her journey includes walking out of sugar addiction by the grace and power of God. She shares honestly and transparently about what it is like to be super morbidly obese and what it takes to turn around and be free. Get your copy in print, kindle or audiobook on Amazon. If you prefer, you can order as a printable eBook from http://teresashieldsparker.com/sweet-grace-order/

"Sweet Grace Study Guide: Practical Steps To Lose Weight And Overcome Sugar Addiction" is designed to be used in conjunction with "Sweet Grace" for personal or group study. It contains chapter studies, activities, action steps and a covenant. Get your copy on Amazon or order a downloadable and printable eBook from http://teresashieldsparker.com/guide-order/

"'Sweet Grace' is life changing! A must read! Teresa reveals her vulnerability in this book that empowers one to join the journey, to throw off strongholds and allow our Creator to heal us and walk in His favor! This is the greatest, most honest book I have every read!"

—Amazon Customer Review

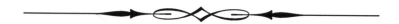

"We have become His poetry, a recreated people that will fulfill the destiny He has given each of us, for we are joined to Jesus, the Anointed One. Even before we were born, God planned in advance our destiny and the good works we would do to fulfill it."

Ephesians 2:10 TPT

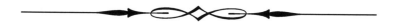